" *Whether you're looking for deep relaxation, stress reduction, or spiritual transformation, you're in good hands with yoga master and nondual psychotherapist Richard Miller, whose wise, warm-hearted, accessible instruction in the time-honored practice of Yoga Nidra has the power to guide you all the way home!"* —STEPHAN BODIAN

Author of *Meditation for Dummies* and *Buddhism for Dummies*, former editor-in-chief of *Yoga Journal*

" *Richard Miller's book on Yoga Nidra makes an enormous contribution to our understanding of this most ancient practice. In a sea of new and often empty publications, this book deserves a place on the bookshelf of any yoga practitioner, be they beginner or teacher. Richard's warmth and radiant presence, so familiar to his student's and colleagues, rings through in every page."* —DONNA FARHI

Author of *Yoga Mind, Body & Spirit* and *Bringing Yoga to Life*

"*Richard Miller is one of this generation's most important teachers of nondual wisdom. Seekers of all kinds will be grateful for this collection, because it is saturated with his beautiful voice, and with the echo, too, of the great voices of his teachers—Jean Klein and Swami Satchidananda. Richard's teaching is both soothing and invigorating—reminding us that in our true nature we are already free, enlightened, and awake. Reminding us that in any moment we could savor Divine presence. For me, simply hearing this view in his graceful words profoundly changes where I stand in relationship to my experience.*

In this collection, Richard brings us the practice of Yoga Nidra with a sophistication and power that it has not previously known in the West. Yoga Nidra is in so many ways the perfect tool for his nondual teachings, and his practices are absolutely delicious—simple, deep, and transformative. Like all authentic spiritual work, these practices produce fruit from the very beginning. They require only presence, and as such represent both the path and the goal of nondual practice." —STEPHEN COPE

Senior Scholar in Residence, Kripalu Center for Yoga and Health; Author of *Yoga and the Quest for the True Self* and *The Wisdom of Yoga*

YOGA NIDRA

Richard Miller, Ph.D.

YOGA NIDRA

The Meditative Heart of Yoga

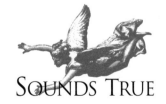

SOUNDS TRUE

Sounds True, Inc.
Boulder CO 80306

© 2005 Richard Miller

Permission to use quotes from Wei Wu Wei, Open Secret,
Hong Kong University Press, Hong Kong, 1982 by:
Sentient Publications, LLC.
1113 Spruce Street
Boulder CO 80302
303-443-2188
www.sentientpublications.com

Published 2005
Printed in Korea

ISBN 1-59179-379-3

Library of Congress Control Number 2005932738

"A single word is sufficient to reveal the truth."
—SHÊN HUI

Gratitude to Laura Cummings and Jean Klein
for keeping the word alive ...

TABLE OF CONTENTS

Acknowledgments

Gratitude to Anne, Jennie, and Sean for living with me in the word; to Nancy Rogers and Tami, Alice, Chad, Nancy, Joe, and everyone else at Sounds True for their help in bringing this book into your life; and to the students, clients, and teachers I've worked and studied with over the decades who have helped me realize the truth of this precious teaching.

Introduction: The Open Secret

When we dwell in the pleasures of our senses, attractions to further pleasures arise. From attraction comes attachment, the desire for possession that leads to passion and burns into anger. Passion and anger cloud judgment and lead to confusion, the inability to learn from past mistakes and the failure to choose between what is wise and what is unwise. This is the path of separation. But when we move in the world of the senses, yet keep our senses in harmony, free from attachment to attraction or aversion, we rest in the wisdom heart of our True Nature, the true equanimity of Being, in which all sorrow and suffering cease.[1]

I was first introduced to the rudiments of Yoga Nidra in 1970, during my first ever Yoga course. At the end of my first lesson, after slowly performing an exquisite sequence of asanas that heightened sensitivity to every part of my body, our instructor led us through *Shavasana*, the traditional yogic pose for inducing deep relaxation while lying completely still on the floor. The instructor expertly guided us into being conscious of sensations throughout our body, as well as to opposing experiences such as warmth-coolness, agitation-calmness, fear-equanimity, sorrow-joy, and separation-oneness. I was invited to rotate my attention through the sensations elicited by pairs of opposites until I was able to embody these opposing experiences with neither attachment nor aversion to what I was experiencing.

I drove home that evening feeling totally relaxed and expansively present. For the first time in years, I felt free of all conflict, radiantly joyful, and attuned with the entire universe. I experienced life as being perfect just as it was and felt my self to be a spacious, non-localized presence. Instead of my usual experience of being in the world, I was having a non-mental experience of the world being in me; similar to experiences I had known as a child.

This experience continued to resonate and left a longing in me to consciously awaken into and fully abide as this sense of presence. It awoke in me the strong desire to deeply understand the art of Yoga and especially the process of Shavasana, which I would later learn as Yoga Nidra. My yearning would eventually lead me to study with some of the most renowned teachers in the world; I became a teacher of Yoga and an adept in the application of Yoga Nidra through years of practice and by guiding thousands of students in its process during innumerable group classes, individual sessions, workshops, and meditation retreats.

During that first Yoga class, I recovered a secret that I now know is open to everyone who is interested in finding true peace of mind, equanimity that remains undisturbed, free of circumstance or situation. And I know that if I can realize it, so can you. The key to inner peace is not some impenetrable secret. While seemingly obscure, it is actually in plain sight and readily available to you—an "open secret." Let Wu Wei Wu explain.

The old Masters were fond of a little joke. One of them might say that the Buddha had a secret, but that Mahakashyapa let it out. Mahakashyapa, you may remember, was the bodhisattva to whom the Supreme Vehicle, chiefly represented by Ch'an and Zen today, is attributed. He it was who understood the famous sermon when the Buddha held up a flower and spoke no word. Then one Master would remark that only as long as you do not understand, is it a secret. And, indeed, do not all mysteries and miracles only appear so, in so far as we may not understand how they arise or occur? Then another might add that once you do understand, it is Mahakashyapa not keeping the secret. Therefore a secret is only something that people in general do not understand and Mahakashyapa not keeping the secret was the real secret of the Buddha. Thus the secret that is not kept secret is what is meant by an Open Secret.[2]

Most of us know the kind of fragile peace that is easily disturbed by the onslaught of daily life. Through the exquisite practice of Yoga Nidra, I discovered an unshakable equilibrium that is present under all circumstances and situations. If it weren't, it wouldn't be real peace. I know that this is true peace because I've tested it over many years in my daily life: in my job, in the marketplace, and in family life. And we're all aware that the true test of inner peace comes not in the meditation hall, but in our daily life and relationships. Yoga Nidra revealed to me the peace of *Presence, Being,* and *Equanimity* that remain steadfast and true during even the most intense and difficult times of physical pain, interpersonal conflict, and current events. I've uncovered it. I've tested it. Now it is my heartfelt desire to share it with you.

THE ORIGINS OF YOGA NIDRA
The origin of Yoga Nidra can be traced back to ancient Eastern teachings of Yoga and *Tantra* (Sanskrit: *tan*——extending everywhere), which are a vast array

of techniques designed to extend our understanding in order to overcome our mind's penchant to divide unitive True Nature into separate objective parts. Tantra and Yoga are not concerned with philosophical intellectualism or second-hand information. These teachings are concerned with firsthand knowing of who we actually are, where we stand free of psychological, cultural, and philosophical conditioning in the truth of what actually is.[3] Various yogis have revitalized the practice of Yoga Nidra throughout the past half century, most notably through the teachings of Swami Sivananda and his various disciples such as Satyananda Saraswati of the Bihar School of Yoga, Swami Satchitananda of Integral Yoga, and Swami Vishnudevananda of the Sivananda Yoga Vedanta Center; Swami Rama of the Himalayan Institute and his direct disciple, Swami Veda Bharati of the Swami Rama Sadhaka Grama; and Sri Brahmananda Saraswati (Rammurti S. Mishra) who was an initiate of the Radhaswami School of Surat Shabd Yoga, among others.[4]

I was introduced to the actual term, Yoga Nidra, through the teachings of Swami Satyananda Saraswati in his many literary offerings, especially his book entitled *Yoga Nidra*. Over the years I've had the privilege of studying with many renowned spiritual teachers who have helped me directly and indirectly refine this exquisite art of meditative inquiry through both my studies in psychology and spirituality.[5]

Through Yoga Nidra, I discovered a profound process that teaches us how to carefully and systematically investigate the nature of our beliefs that define our personal identity and differentiate the world around us into separate objects. For instance, we believe that we are solid and separate and that there is an external world that exists independently of us. But we may never have deeply examined the actual reality of these beliefs. During Yoga Nidra, we investigate our actual experience so that we can understand the nature of who we actually are and what the world really is. Yoga Nidra helps us investigate and dispel the roots of our conditioning that underlie our misperceptions of reality. Yoga Nidra dissolves the obstacles that stand in the way of our leading an authentic life of purpose and meaning, and, for those who are interested, it can awaken us into living an enlightened life of self-realization as our True Nature.

USING THIS BOOK AND CD

In this book and the accompanying CD, I share with you the basic steps of Yoga Nidra, what each step leads to, some of the interim benefits that you will realize along the way, as well as the ultimate discovery that Yoga Nidra reveals. At its minimum, Yoga Nidra will lead you to experience profound relaxation, the release of chronic stress, restful sleep, resolution to many of your life's conundrums, and a greater sense of harmony in your daily life and relationships. In its ultimate revelation, Yoga Nidra points directly to your True Nature, to peace that is beyond description and is your birthright. This peace is not an empty promise or only for a selected few, but is present and available to you right now.

I take great comfort in sharing this delicious practice with you. For me it has withstood the test of time and delivered its promise, and I trust that it will do the same for you. I believe that there is good reason why Yoga Nidra has found its way into your life in this moment. I pray that the practice of Yoga Nidra will be, as it has been for me, your companion for life. It's a trustworthy ally through thick and thin.

I suggest you read this book in its entirety before proceeding to the CD. Orienting your mind to the underlying perspective of Yoga Nidra allows your mind and body to relax as you listen to the actual practice sessions. That said, if you are a person who doesn't like reading manuals, then by all means, dive into the practice. Firsthand experience is the best teacher. But after using the CD, do come back to this text in order to deepen your understanding, which will enable you to obtain maximum advantage from each practice session. I do advise, however, before listening to the CD, that you read through the segment entitled "Setting the Stage" at the end of this introduction so that you can derive maximum benefit from your first experience with Yoga Nidra.

What's in the Book

Chapter One provides an orientation to the perspective of Yoga Nidra. Reading about Yoga Nidra is a bit like reading a description of sugar before you've ever tasted such a treat. The actual taste is beyond words. But I have learned that understanding helps the mind relax and allows us to plunge more deeply into the experience. Keep in mind that Yoga Nidra is not a philosophy. It is a series of experiments you engage in to discover the living truth about yourself and the world. In the final analysis, the proof is in the tasting.

Chapter Two is an overview of the stages of Yoga Nidra, which are presented as actual practice sessions on CD. The CD is set up so that you can work with one or more of these stages of Yoga Nidra, depending upon your need of the moment.

Final reflections on Yoga Nidra are presented in Chapter Three.

The final items in this book will help you further refine your practice of Yoga Nidra. After you've listened to the CD several times, make a copy of the Yoga Nidra Worksheet on pages 73–78 and fill it in with the emotions, beliefs, images, and so on that are specific to you, so that you can personalize your practice within a particular mini-session of Yoga Nidra. Yoga Nidra should never be mechanical. You want the practice to be alive and meaningful. You will learn to adapt the practice to suit your individual needs respecting your gender, age, cultural background, and stage of life. Keep in mind the adage, *"Make the practice your own."*

The References section provides resources for further studies that will provide continuing support for your practice of Yoga Nidra. Why reinvent the wheel? Take advantage of those who have come before you. We have much to share in our journey together.

The Enclosed CD

The first practice on the CD comprises a series of five mini-sessions, each representing a stage of Yoga Nidra. You can listen to an individual mini-session by itself, or flow through them all as a series that make up one entire practice of Yoga Nidra. As you become adept in your practice, you may wish to engage in only one or two mini-sessions to address an existing issue. At other times, you will enjoy flowing through the entire practice.

Yoga Nidra can be performed in a matter of seconds, a few minutes, or it can be an in-depth practice lasting an hour or more. Gandhi practiced Yoga Nidra on the train between speaking engagements. Swami Veda Bharati has used Yoga Nidra to learn a new language overnight. I've used it with students and clients to help them prepare for surgery and solve conundrums and interpersonal issues. Others have used Yoga Nidra to dissolve their fear of flying, resolve past traumas, and obtain restful sleep. And some of us have used Yoga Nidra to inquire into the mystery of life and awaken to our True Nature as Unqualified Presence.

The second practice on the CD is an integrated session of Yoga Nidra that you can listen to many times over. Multiple layers of understanding are imbedded within both Practice One and Two. This CD is designed so that you can return to it time and again over many years, gaining greater understanding and benefit with each practice. I have heard from innumerable students after they have listened to the same session countless times, *"I never heard that before!"*

SETTING THE STAGE

Before beginning your first practice on the CD, please read the following guidelines, which will help make your first sojourn into this wondrous land of Yoga Nidra a fruitful journey.

- Find a quiet place to practice.It's important to practice Yoga Nidra in a room where you can be on vacation, away from external distractions. Think of this room as your personal sanctuary where you are on temporary retreat.
- Turn off the phone. Let your spouse and children know that you're not to be disturbed. When your support system helps you maintain your sacred Yoga Nidra retreat, they will witness the marvelous benefits that practice brings to your life. They will want their own retreat time for Yoga Nidra, too.
- Wear comfortable clothing. Clothing that doesn't constrict circulation or cause discomfort while you practice is best.
- Lie on a comfortable surface, preferably a soft rug or mat. I caution you against using your bed because your subconscious mind associates bed with sleep. While Yoga Nidra mimics sleep, you want to remain alert throughout its practice. When possible, practice in a room other than where you sleep.

Yoga Nidra may also be practiced in a sitting position on a comfortable chair or cross-legged on the floor. When sitting, keep the spine straight and the lower back in its normal concave position. Your knees should be lower than the rim of your pelvis, which enables your back to be upright and comfortable. Whether prone or sitting, keep your forehead, chin, and eyes lowered so that your gaze is toward the floor, rather than the wall. When chin, forehead, and eyes move up, thinking engages. When chin, forehead, and eyes are soft and down, thinking abates. During Yoga Nidra, you want soft eyes so that you are gazing out through the eyes of the heart instead of your mind.

- Cover your eyes with an eye bag or soft towel. Keeping light out soothes the brain.
- If you're lying down, place a rolled towel, blanket, or bolster under your knees. Bending the knees relaxes the lower back and allows your body to be totally supported by the floor.

Keep in mind that, ultimately, I want you to have the mental freedom to practice Yoga Nidra anywhere, in any room, on any surface, under all circumstances, dressed any way that you are. When you are oriented in the correct understanding of Yoga Nidra, nothing need stand in the way of your practice.

Welcome Discomfort, Emotions, Memories, and Your Natural State of Being

Discomfort arises.

But discomfort needn't disturb. Your body is a guesthouse and Yoga Nidra teaches you how to invite every imaginable guest in for "tea and conversation." When discomfort arises, don't try to adjust it away. First, receive and welcome it in as a messenger. Inquire as to what its message is. Sometimes discomfort simply wants to whisper something in your ear and then go on its way. At other times it may want you to adjust your body. Observe your tendency to react—your propensity to jump away from experience. Yoga Nidra is a path of *welcoming* where you are learning to meet, greet, and welcome everything that life brings to your table. Only then will you uncover your innate clarity, right action, and peace of mind.

Emotions and memories do arise.

There are times in Yoga Nidra where you will even seek out emotions and memories and invite them into your guesthouse for "tea and conversation." You possess an innate intelligence that knows exactly what to do in every situation that life brings to your table. When you are willing to be with "this" moment "now," your intrinsic resources are always nearby, ready to acknowledge and engage right action. Fear is always about the future, and reactivity about the past. Right action resides in the "now." Yoga Nidra is a practice that reveals and teaches you how to live in the now so that you can access your native intelligence and inborn ability to respond appropriately to every situation.

Open to Being.

Yoga Nidra reveals that your body, mind, and the entire universe live in you, in your awareness. During practice, you may experience an expansion beyond the confines of your body, which can make you feel like you're having an out-of-body experience. But, no matter how far out you expand, aren't you always "here" as the witness of your experience? Yoga Nidra helps you inquire as to who this witness is, this "I" that you take yourself to be. When you realize True Nature, pure *Being*, you recover your primal memory that your "real body" is everywhere, infinitely expanded. You realize that the entire universe is your body. Then there's no such thing as an out-of-body experience because there's nowhere to go where you aren't already. You're always here, which is everywhere. Life is a paradoxical mystery, and Yoga Nidra hands you the key that unlocks the mystery that is your life and this world.

Consult your resources.

You're never alone. Resources are available to assist and support you at every turn of the road of Yoga Nidra. See the Resources and References sections for books, articles, tapes, people, and places to contact for support and further study. When you're ready, go on retreat where you can learn Yoga Nidra to its fullest extent, where you can practice in community with like-minded people who share your interest of self-understanding and enlightened living. Remember, at any given time and day, thousands of people around the world are practicing with you. You're always in good company when you practice Yoga Nidra.

Yoga Nidra is a time-honored, re-educational process that teaches you how to blend profound relaxation with innate wisdom into every moment of your waking life. The practice of Yoga Nidra leads to sweeping changes within your mind and body, as well as in all of your interpersonal relationships. It's a fundamental resource for transforming your physical health as well as reshaping your personal, interpersonal, and professional relationships. Please understand that Yoga Nidra is not hypnosis, but rather the deepest and most profound but very natural state of meditation. It enables you reconnect to your deepest, most intimate, and relaxed receptivity of intuitive spontaneous intelligence. And it is simple to learn and easy to practice, and a tool that you can use throughout your lifetime.

CHAPTER
ONE

The Marvelous World of Yoga Nidra

IT'S EARLY MORNING, and you're waking from a dream. You can just as easily fall back into the dream images as wake up to answer the call of nature. You'd like to stay here, wouldn't you, in this peaceful twilight state of deliciousness. So you linger here, resting in this delightful state of equilibrium that exists between waking and sleeping, where all problems seem far away. And while you're here, quite unexpectedly, an insight comes. Suddenly it's all very clear, isn't it? When you went to sleep the night before you were in the middle of a conundrum, but now you know what to do, the action you need to take. And you've experienced this before, haven't you. Somehow, mysteriously, while absorbed in this twilight equanimity, insights spontaneously appeared; solutions arrived unbidden, and problems dissolved. How marvelous! How wondrous! How delightful! Welcome to the magnificent world of Yoga Nidra.

WHY YOGA NIDRA

Yoga Nidra is an ancient sacred yogic process of meditation that can be practiced for countless reasons: to induce profound relaxation in your body and mind, eliminate stress; overcome insomnia; solve personal and interpersonal problems; resolve trauma; and neutralize and overcome anxiety, fear, anger and depression. The process deepens the experience of meditation, making it a lifetime habit; as well as encourages meditative inquiry in order to unravel the mystery of life and answer such questions as: "Who am I?" "Why am I?" "What is all of this?" and "What is enlightenment?"

During Yoga Nidra, you enter a profound state of receptive relaxation, all the while remaining totally aware and alert throughout its process. Yoga Nidra invites your innate intelligence and intrinsic clarity to rise to the surface of your conscious mind, allowing you to uncover and access the wisdom resources of your higher levels of consciousness. Your innate intelligence knows the exact solutions, revelations, and resolutions that you need in order to address all the various issues, problems, questions, and conundrums that you face in your daily life.

It is common for spontaneous physical, psychological, and interpersonal transformational shifts to occur during Yoga Nidra, as negative patterns of conditioning are burned away by the fire of discriminative wisdom that ignites as you tap into your innate inner wisdom, a wisdom so powerful that it easily burns through even the most formidable destructive patterns of physical and psychological conditioning.

During Yoga Nidra, David's body feels tense and his heart is pounding with fear as he recalls an image of his parents fighting, their voices loud, angry, and harsh. He's in his bedroom with the pillow over his head, terrified that his parents are going to kill themselves. He feels alone and unsafe.

Yoga Nidra invites David to welcome in an opposite memory, a time when he feels calm and peaceful, and he finds himself in his bedroom as a little boy, tucked in between clean, white sheets. His parents are kneeling on either side, holding hands across his bed, saying a prayer they have created just for him. He hears them praying, word for word and feels safe, secure and loved.

As an adult, David is locked into the belief that the world is an unsafe place. But now, as he rotates his attention over and again through these opposites of experience, he realizes that he is loved and safe and that his parents love each other even amidst their turmoil. This insight transforms his skewed version of the truth.

Yoga Nidra then invites David to relinquish his memories and bask in these feelings of love, wholeness, and safety. Yoga Nidra is reintroducing David to his innate feeling of Being, of which love, wholeness, and safety are but three natural expressions that were obscured as a result of his early trauma. David arises from Yoga Nidra embodying a sense of inner calm that he never believed possible. David is experiencing how love, wholeness, and safety are not incompatible with anger and fear. True Nature—Being—welcomes all experiences and is love in action.

AWAKENING FROM THE DREAM

Yoga, often inadequately translated as *union*, represents both the action of awakening to, as well as the description of our underlying True Nature or pure Being that is the birthing ground of authentic spontaneity.[6] *Nidra* or *sleep*, on the other hand, is the state in which we are unconscious to True Nature, when we are identified with, and swayed by thoughts and actions that are based on misperception and reactive patterns. Yoga Nidra represents a paradox and is a play on the words "sleep" and "awake" as it means *The Sleep of the Yogi* and implies that the normal person is asleep to their True Nature through all states of consciousness—waking, dreaming, and deep sleep—while the yogi is one who is awake to and knows his or her True Nature across all states, even sleep.

When we sleep, we believe our dream-self and dream-world are real. When we wake up, our dream-world gives way to the waking state, and we recognize that the dream-self and dream-world are actually empty of substance. They are only fabrications and projections of the mind.

During waking consciousness, we perceive the world to be made up of solid and separate objects. We believe that our waking thoughts and the objects around us are real. But, could it be that waking-state thoughts and objects are also fabrications and projections of the mind, as empty of substance as our dream-self and dream-world? Yoga Nidra is the process whereby we explore and discover the truth of this fact.

Usually we have no reason to question the validity of these beliefs. But there is good reason why we should. Yoga Nidra reveals that all dream and waking phenomena—thoughts, emotions, sensations, images, and the world around us—are constantly changing, coming, and going. Everything about our body, mind, and the world is constantly changing, morphing from one thing into another, a mass of swirling, changing sensations, emotions, thoughts, and images.

When we are attached to life being consistent, we feel dissatisfied; we suffer, because life constantly changes. We are constantly searching within this sea of instability for something stable and constant to hold onto. Yoga Nidra reveals that the inner fabric of each of us is deep equanimity or peace that is stable and steady, and when realized, is recognized to be ever-present even in the midst of life's tumultuousness. This is what Yoga Nidra refers to as your fundamental True Nature, your innermost I-ness—deep peace that you know, without a shadow of a doubt, that is always present.

Yoga Nidra teaches you how to inquire into the fundamental nature of your "I" that registers the fact that everything is changing. When we inquire into the who, what, and where of the "I" that is witnessing the smorgasbord of life's changing phenomena, we discover that this "I" that we take ourselves to be is not solid either, but paradoxically, unlike everything else, it isn't changing. Yoga Nidra helps you realize that your True Self, or true I-ness, is an infinite and unqualified spacious Presence of Being in which everything, both waking and dream states, is born, unfolds, and dissolves. With Yoga Nidra, you explore and discover the truth of your True Self, as Pure Being.

I am lying on the floor in Yoga Nidra, feeling contracted, sad, and alone. I gently inquire, "Who is this 'I' that is experiencing these feelings? Are there not two here, these feelings and the 'I' who is feeling them?" Suddenly, an inner shift of perspective occurs. Whereas a moment ago I was 'in' these feelings, now these feelings are 'in me.' I experience myself as spacious awareness in which these feelings are arising.

As I lie here feeling both sadness and spacious awareness, I realize that awareness has been present throughout my lifetime, while feelings come and go within it. Foreground and background abruptly switch as I realize that "I" am Awareness. "I," as Awareness, am not contracted and sad. "I" don't feel limited to this body or to these passing feelings. "I" am the spaciousness within which this body lives. Unexpectedly, I sense a subtle truth and a course of action that I had overlooked. Sadness and contraction dissolve as I contemplate action that appears clear and right. But before springing into action, I want to lie here awhile, basking as pure Being, my true "I." I realize all creativity springs from this source. This is the fountain of youth everyone is searching for and it is always here. How amazing, how astonishingly simple, hidden in plain sight—an Open Secret!

AWAKE AT LAST

When we are truly awake, we are no longer swayed by, or identified with any thought, belief, emotion, sensation, image, action, or changing circumstance. We remain awake as True Nature, no matter the circumstance or situation, because the fundamental essence of True Nature is present across all states of waking, dreaming, and even deep sleep.

Yoga Nidra reveals True Nature by its distinct flavor as unshakable peace, equanimity, compassionate love, discriminative wisdom, and authentic and spontaneous action. When we abide as True Nature, we embody our true humanity and become a *purusha* (Sanskrit: one who dwells in the city of True Nature), a true human being wherein our actions, thoughts, and deeds are in harmony with life and with the people around us, who we now recognize as purushas as well, even though they may not yet be awake to their True Nature.

YOGA NIDRA TAKES YOU BEYOND WAKING AND SLEEPING

During dreamless sleep, we are unaware of the stress, tension, and conflict that we experience during our waking state. In fact, we are totally unaware that we have either a body or a mind. In dreamless sleep, there is total disidentification from body and mind, yet we still exist, for when our mind and body re-awaken we are conscious of having slept deeply without dreaming.

During dreamless sleep, we experience a profound sense of contentment and equanimity, for when we awaken we feel rested and relaxed and can exclaim to others that we had a deep and restful sleep. In dreamless sleep, we abide as our Natural State that lies beyond and is totally disidentified from all stress and conflict. This is why we feel so rested upon awakening. The practice of Yoga Nidra teaches you how to consciously live in and as this Natural State of equanimity even as you go about daily life. Abiding in and as True Nature enables you to live through anxiety, tension, and conflict without losing your deep peace and equanimity. Yoga Nidra sensitizes you to recognize your inner light of clarity, which is always present as an expression of True Nature that is constantly revealing your path of right understanding and right action during even your most difficult and challenging circumstances.

RIGHT ACTION

Yoga Nidra teaches you how to recognize and disidentify from your core negative beliefs and habit patterns, which hinder and cripple you from leading a truly contented life free from dissatisfaction and suffering. Dissatisfaction and suffering (Sanskrit: *duhkha* = dissatisfaction, suffering) arise when you mentally attach to expectations and outcomes that are other than what life is offering. When we accept life as it is, dissatisfaction and suffering cease, and we learn to deal with reality on its own terms, rather than through what our mind desires.

When we accept life, we realize that every situation is paired with its perfect response of right action that when engaged, leads us to experience a sense of perfection in each moment. This can be startling to the mind when first encountered, but when you truly accept each moment and embody its perfectly paired response through right action, you will experience wonder, delight, and astonishment at how perfectly orchestrated every moment is.

As our beliefs, assumptions, expectations, and misperceptions dissolve, we abide more and more in authenticity, which opens the door to glimpses of our True Nature as pure Being or Presence, which is the underlying source of authentic living. Yoga Nidra awakens us into the realization that we are not limited and finite as we mistakenly thought we were. We discover, instead, that we are Vastness that is infinite, joyous, loving, kind, compassionate, and always present, even in the midst of the greatest difficulty. When we live our Vastness, we discover that validation comes directly from True Nature, not from external authorities. We recover our gyroscope of internal stability, which naturally arises from True Nature that cannot be shaken or disturbed by inner or outer events, nor swayed by the opinions of others.

Yoga Nidra does not ask us to believe or disbelieve this or for that matter, anything. Rather, it invites us to investigate what we assume to be true through a series of experiments or self-inquiries so that we may relinquish what we have been told and come to our own first-hand understanding about the nature of reality, the world, and ourselves. Yoga Nidra is, therefore, not a philosophy, but a way of living life from firsthand, rather than second-hand information. It's a process we engage in to heal from misperception, anxiety, and fear into equanimity, stability, and love. Here is Mary's experience during a particular Yoga Nidra.

Fear comes thundering in like the roar of the airplane I imagine I am sitting in. My body is drenched in cold sweat, heart pounding, gripped in terror. Every bump and sound of takeoff fuels my fear that something's wrong; this airplane is going to crash! I lay here trembling with fear, body shaking. Then I search for an opposite experience and recall my mother rocking me in her arms. Tranquility and peace fill my body, replacing the fear of a moment before. As I bring together these two opposites of fear and tranquility, suddenly I feel free of both. Instead I feel myself as spacious, open equanimity, which transcends both my emotions of fear and peace. I feel unexpectedly liberated, free in a way I could never have imagined. Yoga Nidra has taken me beyond my feeling separate and introduced me to a realm where I feel one with the universe.

And what has happened about my fear of flying? Recently, while flying east, guess what? No fear! Rather than feeling terrified of the plane, the plane feels like an extension of me. Who "I" am has expanded to include the airplane and the space all around me. A couple of bumps cause a slight contraction, but no upwelling of fear like before. How amazing and what a relief to feel at ease inside an airplane. I am grateful. Yoga Nidra has relieved me of this terrible fear and opened me to a new sense of freedom and oneness with the universe that I could never have imagined possible.

EVERY "THING" IS COMPRESSED SPACE

We have been taught to believe that the physical world is real and solid. But is this so? The mind says it is. Familial and cultural beliefs say that it is so. But when we actually investigate the solidity of any object, we find only vast space. Solidity gives way to molecules; molecules give way to atoms; atoms give way to electrons, which give way to quarks, which give way to energy, which gives way to empty spaciousness. When we truly inquire, the solidity that was here a moment before dissolves. We discover for ourselves that matter is actually only compressed space, devoid of solidity.

Are we separate from what we observe? The mind says, "Yes." But when we observe something, we influence what is being observed because we are not separate from what we are observing.[7] Our belief in separation is actually an illusion that dissolves in the light of true inquiry.

THE EGO-I IS AN AFTERTHOUGHT

We believe in the reality of our ego-I as a separate and distinct entity. Yet when we inquire to find the location of this "I," we find neither location nor solidity. We discover that the ego-I is actually an afterthought, rather than a point of independent will and initiation. Willfulness remains, yet we discover that true "I-ness" is not separate from the spacious Being in which it and everything else arises. I, you, and every "thing" are actually one, not two.[8] This is how one friend describes her experience of Being True Nature.

Every day I live a fresh reprieve from being somebody, without reference to my "former life." It is beautiful and a surprise all the time. There is no discipline, except listening, which is completely outside being reductive or positive. Listening brings this mind to a halt, to its real use. I feel overwhelmed and brought to my knees by it, yet without any sense of diminution. It is astonishing that all of this happens without struggle, nor giving up any "thing."

From the very beginning there has been total paradox when I feel something; what Jean Klein calls the "absence of the absence." I was in the grocery store late one evening when anonymity seems that much easier. There came a moment when the body felt overwhelmingly transparent; a feeling of well-being beyond anything physical; a transparency in which the body was wholly missing. I laughed! I would not have been surprised to find that I truly was invisible to others. It is beautiful to be anonymous. If only everyone knew what this really meant. It is indescribable. It makes itself. You need do nothing.[9]

While it is easy to prove that matter is actually empty spaciousness, that we are not separate from the objects around us, and that the "I" is a fictitious entity without substance, unless we find a way to embody these understandings, they remain intellectual formulations that have no substantive impact on our lives. Scientists who make these incredible discoveries go home at night to their families as if they've discovered nothing of significance. Our lives don't change just because we've intellectually uncovered the fact that "I" doesn't exist and that our Real Nature is empty spacious Being that is the Source of everything. Talking schools of nondualism have existed for millennium. What we're after is firsthand experience that deeply impacts our daily life and significantly changes our negative beliefs and destructive habit patterns.

FIRSTHAND KNOWING

Yoga Nidra insists that intellectual insight give way to heartfelt experiential firsthand understanding. It is one thing to understand facts conceptually. Yoga Nidra beckons you to understand them as your actual embodied experience. Living embodied wisdom frees you from anxiety, fear, and doubt, replacing them with equanimity and an inner gyroscope of unshakable stability.

During Yoga Nidra, we directly face all the changing movements of the body, mind, senses, and the world around us while we undertake simple and direct inquiries. We believe that "I am a separate entity distinct from all others." During Yoga Nidra, we inquire, "Is this true? What is life like when I believe that this is true? What is it like when I don't take this to be true?"

We believe we are a body and when the body dies, we die. We inquire, "Is this true? Am I this body or is it that this body exists in my awareness?" And, if this is so, "Who am I as this awareness?" When we experience anxiety or fear we inquire, "Am 'I' afraid or is it that fear is arising in me?" We ask, "Who or what is this awareness in which fear, anxiety, and depression are arising?" When we are stuck in negative thought patterns we inquire, "If this thought is a movement in 'me,' who, what, and where is this 'I-ness'?"

In order to truly answer these questions and discover unshakable equanimity and the unqualified Presence of Being, we must relinquish our secondhand beliefs based on the testimony of others. Yoga Nidra offers you simple but exquisite tools to gain firsthand knowledge of who you are and how the universe really works. Only then can you be your own authority, free from the tyranny of "shoulds" and the opinions of others, a light unto yourself.

WITNESSING

When we struggle to change what is, into what we believe should be, we invite stress, tension, and conflict into our life. Our constant struggling to change our inner and outer world is a movement born in conflict that creates division. The impossibility of resolution that is inherent in this struggle leads us to feel chronically tense, tired, confused, and stressed. Paradoxically, it is only when we accept our situation, as it is, that we are able to gain insight that allows us to move into new ways of being and responding. Acceptance, however, doesn't mean resignation, which is still a stance of defense against truly accepting what is.

Yoga Nidra teaches you how to be aware of and experience the ever-changing internal and external phenomenon of your life. Yoga Nidra does not ask you to change anything. It asks only that you observe your habitual tendency to want to change things into something other than what they are. True witnessing, which

Yoga Nidra develops, invites clarity of insight and right action as natural and spontaneous outcomes of seeing things as they are. Witnessing, insight, and right action are synonymous with love and compassion, and all are essential qualities of your innate True Nature. Witnessing awareness, which Yoga Nidra reveals, enables you to see all sides of an issue with discriminative wisdom and love. Only through love and discriminative wisdom can you understand and engage truly authentic action that is appropriate to each situation.

DON'T WITHDRAW, DISIDENTIFY

During Yoga Nidra, you learn to disidentify from distracting sensory impressions and habit patterns (Sanskrit: *pratyahara* = restoration of the senses and mind to their natural functioning), which allows you to recognize right action and abide as your innate spacious clarity of Being. The image of a turtle with its head drawn inside its shell is sometimes cited to represent meditation as a drawing away from the world. But Yoga Nidra does not entail withdrawing from the world. You are born with the innate knowledge of how to naturally let go of and resolve stressful situations while remaining in the field of world and action. Yoga Nidra helps restore your natural aptitude to see and respond clearly to each situation you face.

When you are in a room with a loudly ticking clock, you don't need to withdraw from or block out the ticking sound. When you are open to hearing sound without resistance, when you don't fight sound or try to get rid of it, your mind naturally transcends—disidentifies—and goes beyond the sound. While sound continues to be present, it no longer disturbs and distracts the mind. This is how we learn to deal with stressful situations and difficult emotions, thoughts, and sensations.

During Yoga Nidra, we learn to acknowledge and welcome rather than resist and withdraw from every movement that arises in our life and consciousness.

Then letting go occurs naturally and we see our way through to correct understanding and right action. You don't have to be a yogi who lives as a tortoise with your head tucked inside your shell. Yoga Nidra teaches you how to be a yogi who is open to experiencing every movement of life. Your willingness to fully experience life is, paradoxically, what allows you to transcend each experience and live your True Nature in the midst of the circumstances of life.

THE LAW OF AWARENESS

The power inherent in Yoga Nidra is based on the *Law of Awareness.* Whatever you are willing to be with, you go beyond. Sensory impressions and habit patterns that you neither resist nor get involved in expand and pop, dissolve, and disappear, like bubbles rising to the surface of a lake. All movements of sensation, thought, and emotion expand as they come to the surface of your awareness. As they expand, they may appear to be momentarily troublesome. But they are simply seeking the surface, and, when you don't resist, they disintegrate into the spaciousness of awareness. Whatever is allowed to merely be, as it is, in awareness, resolves, dissolves, and disappears. This truth pertains to your every experience.

Sharon is experiencing insomnia and has heard from friends that Yoga Nidra may be a helpful resource. Nothing else has helped up to this point. During her initial session, Sharon learns to delight in the tactile flows of sensation and energy in her body and experiences a great release of tension. During her second session of Yoga Nidra, Sharon learns to welcome, rather than resist, her fear of not being able to sleep at night.

As she invites her fear in for "tea and conversation," she suddenly realizes that she is afraid of falling asleep. An intimate friend of Sharon's unexpectedly died during sleep last year. Sharon unknowingly is harboring the fear that this might happen to her. As Sharon opens to her fear of dying, she feels great relief that it is not sleep that is her concern but the grief of losing a beloved friend. During four subsequent sessions of Yoga Nidra, Sharon welcomes in her grief and realizes that it is an expression of the deep love she feels for her friend. She acknowledges the preciousness of life and welcomes in the actions that she needs to take, and has been postponing, in order to deeply open into her own living. How amazing and unexpected. Welcoming her fear leads Sharon to love, engaged action, and a good night's sleep.

THE MYTH OF SEPARATION

We mistakenly assume that the objects in our awareness are phenomena separate from ourselves. We hear sounds and greet people with the belief that they are "outside," while all the time they are actually "inside" us—inside our awareness, inside as sensory perceptions. And because sensory impressions are not separate from the mind that perceives them, we are not separate from what we perceive. Separation is a mental projection formulated by our senses and mind in order to maintain an ordered inner and outer world of duality.

Experience This Yourself

- Stop reading and listen to the sounds around you for a few minutes. As you listen, notice at first that you attend to a particular sound that is arising from a particular direction.
- After a little while, open to hearing all sounds from all directions simultaneously. Feel how the whole body participates in this global hearing, not just the mind.
- After a few moments, instead of orienting to sound, feel yourself as the awareness in which all sounds are arising. Feel how the thinking mind must stop in order for you to be awareness.
- Abide as awareness even as sounds move in you.
- Now try the same exercise with the eyes and seeing.

In the moment of perceiving, thinking is absent and your thought of being a perceiver is absent. Ego-I is an afterthought that comes 500 milliseconds after perception takes place.[10] The mind, as the ego-I thought, appropriates what is actually a past event and says, "I am having this perception." In so doing, the mind, through the action of thinking, divides perceiving into an apparent two (perceived and perceiver).[11] But the fact remains, in the moment of perceiving, the ego-I is actually absent, and there is only multidimensional perceiving.

Now carry this understanding to its conclusion. When you abide in perceiving without separating from True Nature or Being, separation is absent, even as Being, perceiving, and perceptions continue. Every "thing," every perception, is unfolding in perceiving, and perceiving is unfolding in Being. When you embody this realization, identification with thinking stops (even as thinking continues), the ego-I dissolves, and perceiving reveals Being.

We may be able to repress an experience, but we cannot, ultimately, get rid of it. Everything moves through its unique cycle of birth, growth, decline, and death. Your attempts to control do not change this natural cycle. Better that we allow everything to be just as it is. Things are just as they are, anyway, aren't they?

When you accept and welcome what is, struggling stops, conflict ceases, the restless mind subsides, and your underlying nature as unqualified Being spontaneously shines forth. When you live as Being, you understand that nothing is lacking. Your True Nature *is* complete and resides in equanimity. You don't need to do or obtain in order to "be" happy. You now act not from lack, but from wholeness. You act, not to become, but because it is natural and right to act.

WELCOMING

Refusing creates conflict. What you refuse is repressed into the unconscious, and whatever lives in the unconscious is projected out into the world. When you reject anger you project anger into the world. You judge others because you judge your own actions. When you stop judging "self," you stop judging "other."

Embodying this understanding is powerfully transformative. When we stop trying to change and learn to be aware, magic happens. Awareness is like fire. Fire purifies, and awareness purifies. Fire doesn't judge. It simply burns away the impurities of what is placed within its presence. During Yoga Nidra, we learn to rest in and abide as the fire of awareness. This is the action of *welcoming* all that is, which is founded upon the insight that trying to change what is always fails. When we rest in and as the fire of awareness, we cease trying to be different and are open to the unknown, welcoming without goal or intention.

When we do not accept ourselves as we are or life as it is, we engage in self-hatred. Non-accepting is a form of self-loathing. When we wish our experience to be other than it is, we fight with reality. And reality always wins. The paradox of welcoming is that it leads to spontaneous transformation. When we relinquish our attempts to change the world or ourselves according to some belief about how we think things "should" be, insight and right action spontaneously arise to the surface of awareness. Then you will live in welcoming for its own sake because of the joy and freedom it brings.

David has spent many sessions of Yoga Nidra learning to welcome the myriad sensations, emotions, and thoughts that endlessly pass through his body and mind. David's attention, no longer absorbed in these movements, is now free to turn into and examine welcoming itself. With a few words of encouragement, he begins to discern the difference between being a welcomer and being Welcoming, wherein his sense of being a separate ego-I dissolves and he feels himself as Being, expressing itself as Welcoming.

David later reports that during this session all sense of separation "melted away, and I was absorbed in a great ocean of joy that seemed to be everywhere, and quite independent of any particular experience. I felt myself basking in my own sunshine. My body felt completely disarmed by a sense of boundlessness that took me into itself. I felt an extraordinary aliveness, that the body was alive in me. I felt a bit overwhelmed when I realized the real force of that aliveness was not coming from my physical body. Quite the opposite. Thoughts and experiences continued, but I felt myself to be the aliveness in which they came and went. Actually, let me restate that. I feel myself, even now, to be aliveness in which everything is coming and going."

DAILY LIFE

It is wonderful to bear witness to people from all walks of life awakening to their unqualified Presence through this exquisite practice of Yoga Nidra. And what is equally beautiful is to hear how it is transforming their daily life and relationships. David's glimpse of True Nature continues to saturate his daily life. Problems still occur, but for him nothing seems to diminish the aliveness that he has uncovered. Several months later, David continued his report.

I see clearly now that my daily experiences are discontinuous. My mind's activity obscures the underlying Being. So, in fact, Being is the continuity . . . everything else is completely contingent upon Being. I see the forcefulness with which my mind gets in the way of observation . . . and I am continually being transformed by this seeing. I am completely astonished by the turning into what I really am that is happening on a day-to-day basis in my life. And nothing seems to hinder this from happening. My relationships are completely different now because my relationship to myself is totally different. I would never have thought this possible.

So now let's look into the actual practice of Yoga Nidra and see how it can transform your life, too.

CHAPTER TWO

The Practice of Yoga Nidra

OUR MINDS' NEED consistent training in order to break free of habits that cause tension and conflict and keep us away from our natural state of peace. It is not difficult to resolve conflict when we know what to do. Patient practice brings success and bears its rewards of love, openness, and right action.

SHEATHS OF SEPARATION

Western science and Yoga acknowledge three constantly changing states: the physical, mental, and energetic, which Yoga further divides into six sheaths or bodies (Sanskrit: *kosha* = sheath, body) and one underlying Essence of True Nature that is changeless. Yoga Nidra reveals that aversion and attachment (not wanting what is to be as it is) to any changing state are the driving forces that fuel chronic stress, pain, conflict, anxiety, depression, insomnia, and lack of peace. Yoga Nidra is a process that enables you to find and relinquish your hidden aversions and attachments associated with each of these changing sheaths of phenomena.

Each stage in Yoga Nidra addresses a particular sheath. As you move through the stages, stress, conflict, and constriction melt away, disclosing authentic insight and right action, and uncaused happiness, contentment, and peace that exist independent of all changing states of body, mind, and senses. During an individual session of Yoga Nidra, you work with a particular sheath, several sheaths, or all the sheaths in succession.

Sheaths and Stages of Yoga Nidra
- Stage 1—Physical Body (*annamaya kosha*): Awareness of sensation
- Stage 2—Energy Body (*pranamaya kosha*): Awareness of breath and energy
- Stage 3—Emotional Body (*manomaya kosha*): Awareness of feelings and emotions
- Stage 4—Body of Intellect (*vijñanamaya kosha*): Awareness of thoughts, beliefs, and images
- Stage 5—Body of Joy (*anandamaya kosha*): Awareness of desire, pleasure, and joy
- Stage 6—Body of Ego-I (*asmitamaya kosha*): Awareness of the witness or ego-I
- Stage 7—Natural State (*Sahaj*): Awareness of changeless Being

Keep in mind that sheaths are only conceptual tools used to organize Yoga Nidra in order to practice in a consistent manner. Yoga Nidra does not require that you believe anything. The only requirement is that you practice and discover for yourself the intrinsic healing power of Yoga Nidra.

Each sheath may be likened to a territory we travel to. Upon arrival, we explore and map out the landscape of each sheath, getting to know it, all the while welcoming the various sensations, thoughts, emotions, and images that we encounter along the way. We learn to relinquish our identification with all internal and external movements and just *be* in this moment as it is and as we are. This may be difficult to grasp because you are habituated to identifying with your thoughts, emotions, and sensations. Yoga Nidra affirms, "Stop identifying with your thoughts. Then solutions will appear and conflict and disharmony will dissolve."

STEP ONE—THE SEARCH FOR TRUTH: SETTING YOUR INTENTION

The only way out is to simply observe.   —JEAN KLEIN

Before beginning Yoga Nidra, we often begin with two preliminary steps. In Step One, you assert your intention to give the practice your wholehearted attention. This intention sets the stage for your mind to remain focused and undistracted throughout each session of Yoga Nidra. From this perspective, Yoga Nidra is a form of mindfulness training wherein the mind regains its ability to be one-pointed and undistracted.

The mind is usually many-pointed, constantly distracted and moving in many directions from object to object, never resting for more than a few milliseconds. It is often preoccupied, and identified with innumerable opposites, constantly seeking pleasure and satisfaction while trying to avoid pain and dissatisfaction. Our preoccupation with one pole of various pairs of opposites reinforces our perception of duality and incites conflict, separation, and suffering. From the perspective of Yoga Nidra, identification by the mind with the ever-changing pairs of opposites is the underlying cause of suffering.

As you recognize and abide as Being, your mind learns not to fight with changing experiences and allows them to be as they are. Misperception based on dualistic thinking dissolves, and equanimity is irrevocably recognized even in the midst of everyday living. While pragmatically one-pointedness is a prerequisite, ultimately, the mind does not have to be one-pointed in order for equanimity to be recognized because in reality the equanimity of Being is always present no matter your state of mind or body.

Sleep of the Yogi

During Yoga Nidra, we intentionally enter into a state that approximates sleep, during which dream-like movements spontaneously appear. But unlike sleep, during which the mind unconsciously identifies with these movements, during Yoga Nidra we bear witness to these mental dream-like fragments. We remain aware rather than falling into unconscious identification with them. We learn to live consciously as witnessing Presence that is always awake and full of equanimity even when the body-mind enters into sleep. This is the paradoxical process of being awake while asleep, wherein we recognize our unqualified Presence that exists independent of the body and the mind.

Usually when we fall asleep, our mind identifies with the dream-doer. When the body is awake the mind identifies itself with the awake-doer. When the mind identifies itself as a doer, whether we are awake or sleeping, background Being remains veiled. In Yoga Nidra, the mind's identification with being a doer dissolves and Being moves to the foreground. Ultimately, Being is recognized to be present whether objects are present (as in waking and dream states) or absent (as in dreamless sleep or when the mind stops thinking during waking life).

STEP TWO—DISCOVERING FOOTPRINTS: YOUR HEARTFELT PRAYER

Truth is always here. It is already the case.   —RICHARD MILLER

After acknowledging your desire to remain one-pointed, which is founded upon our love for what is, you move on to Step Two of Yoga Nidra. Here, you locate heartfelt prayers that you hold about loved ones or yourself. These may be prayers of gratitude, love, enlightenment, health, or healing. You welcome these prayers into the foreground of your conscious mind. You don't hold your prayers as future possibilities. Instead, you affirm them in the present tense as existing realities.

Yoga Nidra reveals that we always live in the present moment; for in reality, there is only the timeless now. We may be thinking about the future or the past, but we are always doing so in the present moment. There is only this present moment, the eternal now. When you were in a past moment, your actual experience then was that it was "now." And when you arrive in some future moment, your experience will also be that it is "now." Ask yourself in any moment, *"What time is it?"* and your firsthand experience will always be, *"It's now."* In reality there is only now, which is our actual experience before the thinking mind divides the seamless now into conceptual past and present.

When we position our prayers in the future, we strive for something that will never arrive. So we always phrase prayers in the present tense. Instead of saying "I will be healthy," "I will feel loved," or "My friend will be cured of disease," we affirm, "I am whole, healed, and healthy," "My True Nature is love, which I am in this moment," or "My friend is healed, whole, and healthy." When the future arrives, it will be now. So we acknowledge this fact by making the future reality of our prayers the actuality of this moment and set our prayers in the language and reality that they are true, now. Each prayer must evoke an attitude of gratitude for the truth that it is conveying. So affirm their truth with your entire mind, heart, and body.

I once visited a friend who was undergoing chemotherapy and feeling depressed and hopeless. His prayer for healing was set firmly in the future, so I invited him to rephrase it into the present tense and to feel its truth as he affirmed it. He was shocked at the difference when he stated, "I am whole, healed, and healthy." He realized that in spite of the cancer and his body feeling sick and exhausted, something inside him did feel "whole and healthy" and in no need of healing. As we sat together he had a spontaneous glimpse of True Nature and realized he had never been sick a day in his life. He realized that indeed, "I am whole and healthy in spite of what is happening in my bodymind." It was a remarkable revelation for him, and had a lasting impact on his psychospiritual well-being.

Once your prayers are acknowledged, you set them aside so that you can revisit them at the end of the practice when you are in the disposition of complete openness and can experience your prayers as present moment realities. Living your prayers in this manner opens them to their full potential.

STAGE ONE—PERCEIVING TRUTH: SENSING YOUR BODY

When you come to innocent, unconditioned listening, your body goes spontaneously into deep peace. —JEAN KLEIN

Now that intention and prayer are in place, you begin systematically rotating attention through the *Physical Body (annamaya kosha)* to counteract the physical disturbances that appear when you lose touch with your inherent omnipresent spaciousness. Innocent, unconditioned listening to physical sensation reestablishes your body's innate radiance.[12] Through the simple act of body sensing, you will grow to appreciate your body as a rich source of effervescent feedback that is always pointing back to its innate ground of physical, psychological, and spiritual vitality.

Radiant Omnipresence

You may believe that the skin defines the boundary of your body. But the body is actually a multidimensional vibration that extends infinitely beyond any conceptual limitation of center or periphery. True Nature has neither center nor periphery. It is simultaneously everywhere because it is omnipresent by nature. Unfortunately, we have forgotten this as our lived experience. We have grown numb to the infinite variety of physical sensations that form the radiance that is our body. This is why disease processes can go undetected for months or years before they erupt to the surface of awareness as discomfort or pain. We are usually unaware of the subtle messages that our body is sending as it tries to inform the mind that something is amiss.

Kaleidoscope of Information

When we are unable to perceive subtle body sensations, we must wait for grosser impressions to emerge into awareness. Unfortunately, by the time we recognize these sensations it may be difficult to heal what is ailing the physical or mental body. Yoga Nidra attunes us to the subtle energetic resonances that make up the physical body. As we discern the myriad array of sensation that our body is constantly emitting, we become creative caretakers of this beautiful temple of vibration that is our body.

As you relearn to feel your body as subtle radiant vibration, you gain access to a vast kingdom of feedback that enables you to experience the entire range of messages that your body is constantly providing regarding its current state of physical, psychological, and spiritual health. We've forgotten how to meet, greet, and listen to the messages that the body is constantly sending.

When we don't "hear" its subtle feedback, the body may turn up its volume by providing gross physical and mental symptoms. The good news is that the practice of Yoga Nidra reawakens your innate capacity for hearing even the subtlest cues that the body is sending. Then you will be able to affirm the yogic proverb, "What to the ordinary person feels like a microscopic spec of dust in the eye, to the yogi feels like a large splinter of wood." When you can acknowledge and welcome the body's cues, you will be able to respond with appropriate action long before your body becomes sick. This is only one of many miracles that Yoga Nidra reveals.

The Homunculus

When we rotate awareness through the physical body, we begin and end in a particular order. We begin in the mouth and end in the feet by tracing precise pathways in the body that have been mapped out by Yoga practitioners for thousands of years. Modern neurophysiologists have also explored these pathways using electrodes to probe the precise interconnections between the physical body and the brain. They have mapped out a vast array of nerve fibers that move to and from the cerebral cortex of the brain, which correlate with precise areas in the physical body.

We give special importance to these sensory-enriched areas as we rotate attention through the physical body during the practice of Yoga Nidra. We begin in the mouth, ears, and eyes, move down the neck into the arms, hands, and fingers, then down the torso into the pelvis and into the feet and toes. As we move through the physical body in this manner, we are simultaneously traveling through the homunculus by way of the sensory and motor cortex areas of the brain. By heightening awareness of our physical body, we are able to simultaneously effect a deep relaxation in brain activity, which heightens our ability to be both alert and relaxed at the same time. Yoga Nidra relaxes the mind by relaxing the body and relaxes the body by relaxing the mind.[13]

The Chakras

While Western science provides a map that pinpoints the most sensitive areas of the body according to the sensory and motor cortex, Yoga provides another map that identifies areas of energetic significance, the *chakras* (Sanskrit: energy centers of the body). Often associated with the seven glands and nerve plexuses of the human body, the chakras are extraordinary, complex, interwoven energetic networks (Sanskrit: *sukshma sharira*) that are constantly providing us with exquisite information regarding our physical, mental, and spiritual health.

These Western and Eastern maps help us rotate attention through the body in a systematic manner that ensures a quick and profound relaxation in both body and mind. When we rotate consciousness through the body, practice after practice, we recover the body as radiant expansive vibration that dissolves stress, promotes vibrant health, and reawakens our inborn disposition of nondual Being. Currently, you may only experience your hand as tingling sensation encapsulated by the walls of the skin; through Yoga Nidra, you realize the hand as a vast field of multidimensional vibration extending infinitely in all directions. Body sensing awakens the body as Vastness unfathomable to the mind, unlimited by conceptual boundaries. Ultimately, Yoga Nidra discloses this as the truth concerning all objects. All objects are compressed radiant vibration. And everything, taken together, is radiant Presence, vibrating from Itself to Itself. This you realize through your practice of Yoga Nidra.

Invent Nothing, Deny Nothing

During Yoga Nidra, you learn to pay close attention to the naturally arising phenomena of your body and mind. You neither invent nor deny anything. Yoga Nidra is not a strategy of self-improvement. Listening and welcoming are your tools, and Yoga Nidra is your process for learning how to listen and welcome all that you are and all that life is—without intention for anything to be other than it is.

We have no intention to fight with or go beyond anything that arises. When sensations arise without resistance, they bubble up and dissolve in awareness just like bubbles rising to the surface of a lake. As they dissolve, we perceive the deeper levels that lie below them. What is important is that we neither get involved with nor repress our experiences. In Yoga Nidra, we proceed through a natural progression moving from gross sensation to very refined levels of energy. For instance, we move from perceiving gross body sensation during Stage One of Yoga Nidra, to being aware of subtler movements of energy during Stage Two while working with the Energy Body.

STAGE TWO—CATCHING TRUTH: AWARENESS OF BREATH AND ENERGY

One who understands the breath quickly tastes the ecstasy of liberation.

—GORAKSASHASTRA

Rotating attention through the Physical Body awakens understanding of the body as infinite radiant vibration. As we experience this vibratory field, what at first is perceived as gross sensation, gives way to subtler levels of energy. We begin to naturally experience the subtle *Energy Body (pranamaya kosha)* that animates and gives life to the Physical Body. Our breath is intimately linked to the Energy

Body, and it is here that we become mindful of our breathing, which allows us to transition gracefully into Stage Two of Yoga Nidra, the exploration of the sheath of energy that animates the physical body.[14]

We initially contact and explore the Energy Body by being attentive to our breathing. We join with and follow the breath without interfering. We observe and experience the body "being breathed" through its natural cycles of inhalation and retention and exhalation and suspension. We don't change or alter the breath in any way. We simply note and experience the breath as a spontaneous activity. By attending to the breath, you become conscious of the subtle energies that animate the breath and give life to the physical body.

Breath Counting

As well as following its spontaneous movement, we also spend time counting each breath. Counting is a form of mindfulness or one-pointedness training. We want to develop the mind's ability to remain with a task for as long as is necessary to accomplish it. If we are to succeed in our endeavor, be it bringing an end to insomnia or anxiety, healing the body of a particular disease, accomplishing a work-related task, or awakening to True Nature, the mind needs to possess the ability to remain oriented. Breath counting develops the mind's ability to remain undistracted for as long as an undertaking requires attention.

When counting breaths, you will be distracted by random thoughts. When this occurs, you begin counting anew. You begin again, and again you will lose your focus. Being distracted and refocusing occurs over and over again. This practice of counting is sharpening your mind's ability to remain undistracted for long periods of time. With practice, you will find yourself alert and undistracted even as numerous potentially distracting thoughts arise. Undistracted attention is now available for you to recognize subtler movements of energy in the body.

Sensing and Breathing

You may experience the movement of your breath first as flows of sensation. But with practice, you will be aware of the naturally occurring subtle flows of energy in your body. It is one thing to conceptually understand that the body is energy. Yoga Nidra is a practice that allows you to experientially realize this fact.

For instance, as you listen to the accompanying CD, I will invite you to perform exhalation and inhalation focusing on sensation and energy flows in the left nostril and on the left side of your body. I will then ask you to perform exhalation and inhalation focusing on sensation and energy flows in the right nostril and on the right side of your body. In this way, you integrate the practice of mindfulness through observing the movement of your breath while sensing the energy flows that animate your breath and physical body. At first this may feel impossible, reminiscent of being asked to chew gum, rub your stomach, and pat your head at the same time. In time you will discover, as I have, the wondrous physical, mental, and spiritual clarity that come as a result of doing this simple practice of breath and energy awareness.

STAGE THREE—TAMING TRUTH:
AWARENESS OF FEELING AND EMOTION

Out beyond ideas of wrong-doing and right-doing is a field. I'll meet you there.[15]

—RUMI

As you experience the currents of energy that animate the body, deeper components of feeling and emotion naturally surface into awareness. This is a signal that you have entered the domain governed by the *Body of Feeling and Emotion* (*manomaya kosha*). Here we welcome and invite into awareness naturally arising pairs of opposites of feeling and emotion such as hot and cold, light and heavy, comfort and discomfort, happiness and sadness, anger and calmness, and powerful and helpless. (Tables 1 and 2, and pages 78–81).

Spacious Awareness

Try the following exercise before reading on:

- Be aware for a few moments of sensation in your right hand.
- Then feel sensation in your left hand.
- Now feel sensation in both hands simultaneously.
- Now shift your attention from sensation in your hands, to the spacious awareness in which these sensations are arising.

What happens to your thinking mind when you are aware of both hands simultaneously? Observe how thinking stops, your sense of being a doer, or "me," drops away and awareness expands to encompass the various sensations. When the thinking mind stops, awareness moves foreground, and can more easily be recognized. When you are oriented, sensation is an exquisite pointer to the awareness in which it is arising. While living in this third sheath, we work with opposites of feeling and emotion in the same manner as we worked with sensation in the Physical Sheath and breath in the Energy Body.

The Law of Opposites

When you live identified with the belief of being a separate ego-I, you are governed by the *Law of Opposites* in which all that is seen as positive is held captive by its opposite. Darkness cannot exist without light, or good without evil. Pain cannot exist without pleasure, or conflict without its opposite, peace. Opposites are complementary polarities arising within a unified field of awareness. Opposites are always paired, and our suffering is sustained by our inability to experience and transcend any pair of opposites.

As you explore the Body of Feeling and Emotion, you are playing in fields of opposites where you invite into awareness the myriad array of feelings and emotions that you will likely experience during your lifetime. You can, for instance, welcome the feeling of comfort and then invite its opposite, discomfort, into the body. You then swing back and forth between these two feelings going first to comfort, then to discomfort and back again, until finally you experience both simultaneously. You will do this with naturally occurring feelings such as warmth-coolness, lightness-heaviness, and pleasure-pain. Then you play in the opposites of emotion. You may take the emotions of calmness and peace and then explore their opposites of agitation and anger. Or you may choose the emotions of joy and happiness and then find their opposite in sadness, despair, and hopelessness.

When you work with opposites in this manner, you explore where specific feelings and emotions are experienced in particular areas of the body. For instance, the perineum and legs are often associated with opposites of safety-fear, security-insecurity, and groundedness-ungroundedness. You move back and forth between these pairs of opposites while noting the sensations that arise in their associated areas such as the legs, pelvis, sexual organs, solar plexus, heart, arms, throat, and head.

When you work with the opposites, you are awakening the discriminating insight that every experience, when fully allowed, is both an expression of, as well as a pointer to, your underlying nondual True Nature. Yoga Nidra respects the transformative power that opposites play in sustaining and resolving disease and suffering and how they are utilized for the purpose of enlightenment.

Fearlessness
Repressed and unresolved feelings and emotions, stored in the unconscious,

give rise to physical and mental unrest. There are many feelings and emotions that we do not want to be with. We refuse them when they come uninvited into our environment. When they arise, we move away, often with reactivity and defensiveness.

The process of Yoga Nidra helps us acknowledge, welcome, and accept these pockets of repression and aversion. When so-called "positive" or "negative" emotions rise up, we meet, greet and welcome rather than refuse them. Yoga Nidra teaches us not to be afraid of feeling afraid, not to be insecure about feeling insecure, and not to resist feeling joyous, open, and vulnerable.

When we welcome opposites of feeling and emotion just as they are, they move naturally through their stages of birth, growth, decay, and death, ultimately dissolving back into their home ground of Being. Feelings and emotions are only passing phenomena, naturally occurring movements in the body and mind. Yoga Nidra introduces us to our ground of innate stability that is present whether strong feelings or emotions are present or absent.

In time, with consistent practice, Yoga Nidra helps us recognize that our natural ground of Equanimity is always present through everyday affairs. You will realize that fearlessness pervades your life when you are no longer afraid of feeling fear or joy. When you are open to feeling whatever is present, attachment and aversion no longer control your life and you live the ease of Being, which evokes profound relaxation and clarity in both your body and mind. Judgment loses its grip, and compassionate love of self and other blossoms.

Here is what one participant had to say after a retreat where she was able to engage various feelings and emotions during Yoga Nidra.

Little did I know that hugely embarrassing thoughts and feelings would come up during Yoga Nidra: thoughts about sexuality, unmentionable body parts, all kinds of things one isn't supposed to feel! At least not polite ladies like me! Ha! Richard explained that words in and of themselves were not the issue, but the emotion that the words evoked, like shame and embarrassment. However, even the words themselves were bristling with power and embarrassment, so I had to feel them, otherwise I was censoring myself and not being with my truth. Each time I felt one of these forbidden parts my heart would pound. I was scared. I was embarrassed. But feel them I did. Not feeling them was just too painful. I wondered, "How many forbidden things would I have to feel before I ran out? Is this ever going to end?" So, I spent a lot of Yoga Nidra dealing with these unmentionables. Who said Yoga Nidra is bliss? It felt more like going into battle.

So, what good came of this? As I stayed with the truth of what I was feeling, I felt empowered. I got to practice being with my truth without skirting, without looking away, and it felt liberating. Now I notice that I am more at ease and comfortable with people. Instead of avoiding them, I can look them in the eye without feeling shame or embarrassment. Before I never knew what was the source of my discomfort in being with other people. During Yoga Nidra, rejected parts of myself that made me feel separate, my sexuality, for instance, came knocking on my door saying, "Let me in! I am YOU! Stop rejecting me." So I let these parts in and now I understand what Richard means when he talks about messengers wanting to come in for "tea and conversation." When things that I reject, my very self, come knocking urgently on my door, they ask me to let them in so that I can feel healed, whole, and complete.

Tailoring the Practice to Your Needs

As you become familiar with the process of Yoga Nidra, you will want to tailor the practice specifically to your individual needs. For instance, while preparing to work in the Body of Feeling and Emotion, pick several feelings and emotions that you are having difficulty being with, as well as several that you enjoy experiencing (see pages 79–80 for examples). Pair opposites of feeling and emotion before going into your practice, and then work with them during Yoga Nidra.

For instance, while you are listening to "Practice One: Sensing Feelings and Emotions" on the enclosed CD, replace my words of feelings and emotions with your words so that your practice is creatively structured for your own needs.

The Myth of Separation

Duality is made up of the entire spectrum of opposites and arises within the unified field of True Nature. Duality arises when the senses and mind split nondual Being into separate objects. This is their natural function. It is only when your mind believes that this split is real that difficulty arises. Suffering and conflict co-arise when separation is believed to be real and the only reality that exists. Yoga Nidra is an effective tool for healing this myth of separation. The power of Yoga Nidra, with its focus on welcoming opposites, is based on the insight that, without healing, the root belief in separation, conflict, anxiety, fear, dissatisfaction, and suffering will never be dispelled.

When we experience only one-half of a pair of opposites, for instance, grief versus joy, or shame versus potency, we remain stuck in our experience, unable to move forward. By learning to experience the entire spectrum of opposites of sensation, feeling, emotion, and beliefs (shame and potency, grief and joy), we are able to deconstruct and move beyond limiting beliefs and experiences. Psychological, physical, and spiritual integration unfolds naturally when we cease trying to rid ourselves of our experience and instead open to the full spectrum of opposites.

Ego-Identity Maintains Division

The ego-I is the product of the dividing mind that splits the world into self and other. Ego-identity does not accept the interdependence of opposites; this would mean the end of its separative existence. So the mind, as the ego-I, attaches to and tries to avoid various opposites, which leads to discord and suffering as any attempt to eliminate one pole of opposition only creates conflict.

Meditation based upon the premise that you need to change begins and ends in conflict. Stances that suggest you need to be other than you are promote the belief that there is something wrong with you that needs to be fixed. These stances ultimately fail. These attitudes are a product of the dividing mind. It is only when you welcome every movement of life, grief and joy, shame and potency, sadness and happiness, fear and safety that you are able to go beyond the pairs of opposites and uncover true freedom.

The Tyranny of the Shoulds

The mind inherently identifies with whatever thought, feeling, or emotion is present. And the mind's most deeply held conviction is that of being a separate ego-I. This belief births defensive reactions against perceived threats, which are expressed as, "I [you] should or shouldn't . . ." The tyranny of these "shoulds" is the mind's way of maintaining an unstable equilibrium, based on its tendency to hold only one pole position of any pair of opposites. For example, holding on to guilt or shame prevents its resolution in potent, responsive action. Holding onto despair prevents its resolution with joy. Holding on to one-half of any pair of opposites maintains the mind's belief in being a separate ego-I.

Welcoming Opposites

Yoga Nidra emphasizes welcoming the entire content of consciousness, allowing each experience of psychic material to arise complete with its attendant movements of sensation, emotion, and belief. As you engender the attitude of welcoming, defensive strategies are uncovered. Welcoming evokes insight into self-defeating patterns that are based on refusing to be with confusing, disorienting, overwhelming, or threatening sensations, feelings, emotions, and beliefs.

Welcoming is not an action undertaken by an ego-I. Welcoming is an essential movement of your innate nondual Being. While at first you may believe that "you" are the one "doing" welcoming, during Yoga Nidra, you will recognize that Welcoming is your True Nature, what you are always Being.

As opposites are welcomed, attention is freed to inquire into the form and substance of Welcoming itself, and the quality of Equanimity that it brings. Then the emphasis shifts from focusing upon the changing content of consciousness, to the nature of welcoming Presence. What has been background, Presence, moves foreground, becoming both witness and witnessed, subject and object.

STAGE FOUR—RIDING TRUTH HOME: AWARENESS OF THE BODY OF INTELLECT

Investigate the nature of mind and it will disappear. Thoughts change, but not you.
—RAMANA MAHARSHI

As we explore pairs of emotional opposites, beliefs, images, and entire stories spontaneously arise. This is the signal that we have entered the *Body of Intellect (vijñanamaya kosha)*. Here, beliefs, images, and memories emerge that are associated with unconscious personal, collective, and archetypal forces. Beliefs and images that arise vary across a wide spectrum from positive thoughts, images, and memories to very dark and negative ones. You may experience beliefs and scenes that evoke fond and loving memories or encapsulate chaos, destruction, and death. As before, we intentionally pair positive with negative beliefs and images and move back and forth between the pairs of opposites until we are comfortably capable of being with either side with neither attachment nor resistance. Then we invite both to be present simultaneously. Here they resolve into a higher order of understanding that you may have never considered.

During Yoga Nidra, we learn to welcome every possible experience that life brings to our table while we live in the understanding that everything is a facet of the diamond that is True Nature. The mind may resist this understanding by exclaiming, "How could *this* be a facet of True Nature?" This is the way the mind divides what is One into the many and maintains separation through the Law of Opposites. But remember, every situation is paired with its perfect response. Your mind's resistance falls away when you recognize truth. Then right action is always revealed. When we don't resist opposites, when we welcome each moment and engage action that our heart knows is true, opposites always resolve into the deeper truth that they veil. And when we are oriented, truth is always an exquisite pointer to its home ground of True Nature.

Messengers of Truth

Our beliefs and expectations contain opposites of positive and negative. The expectation that I hold that you will show up on time for our appointment allows me to go about my week in a relaxed and organized manner. This is the positive aspect. If you consistently show up late, or constantly miss appointments, I will feel irritated, which is the messenger informing me that I am running into an expectation that I need to clarify. This is positive. The negative occurs if I become righteously indignant with you for "breaking your agreement" as a result of my mind clinging to the expectation that you "should" show up on time each week. Then, I am blaming you for *my* expectation. It is my mind's clinging to expectations that cause irritation to arise, not your behavior.

During Yoga Nidra, as you live in the Body of Intellect, you learn to welcome and explore all negative and positive beliefs with the understanding that any belief divides and limits when you attach to or refuse one pole of opposites. By learning to listen to your opposites of thoughts, beliefs, expectations, and images, you are learning to welcome them as messengers that are always pointing you to truth and right action.

As you listen to the accompanying CD, I invite you to bring in your personal beliefs and their paired opposites that you find when you work with the Yoga Nidra Worksheet on pages 73–78. Beliefs can be a simple expectation such as "You should show up on time," or long term attitudes such as, "I'm a fake," "It's dangerous to express my real feelings," "I'm flawed, worthless, and unlovable," "No one listens to me," or "I always know what's right." When you locate a belief, pair it with its opposite. "I'm unlovable" might be paired with "I love and value myself." And "I'm not good enough" might be paired with "I am always doing the best that I know how in every moment."

During Yoga Nidra, Susan is learning to welcome sensations of shame and lack of energy without attaching to or pushing them away. After a few minutes, she seeks out their opposites, remembering a time when she is five years old, her body full of energy and vitality. She welcomes these feelings without attaching to them. Then Susan begins rotating her attention between these opposing experiences of shame and potency. After several rotations she experiences these opposites simultaneously. Integration is taking place as she experiences her generative, potent playfulness even as she is experiencing the powerlessness and confusion that led to feeling shame and overwhelm. Susan later reports feeling an energetic shift as she is holding the opposites that enable her to recapture and embody her potency and aliveness even as she experiences the memories that led to her feeling shame. After Yoga Nidra Susan radiates a newfound confidence and sense of loving compassion toward her self and her memories.

It is important to match beliefs with their accompanying images and memories. During Yoga Nidra we intentionally bring in disquieting memories and images in order to recover our innate capacity to be with whatever life brings to our table. We cannot stop the tumultuous waves of turmoil and confusion, but we can learn to sail through them. The practice of Yoga Nidra is your sailboat, instructor, and sailing lesson all rolled into one. Be willing to be surprised. You will fall into delight, wonder, and astonishment with the creative resolutions that True Nature evokes.

Essential Qualities of True Nature

During this phase of Yoga Nidra, we may also invite, welcome, and embody essential qualities of True Nature such as gratitude, love, and compassion (see the lists of opposites on pages 79–80). For instance, you may embody the quality of transpersonal will by surrendering into the feeling evoked by the phrase, "Not my will; Thy will be done." Or you may invite in the feeling of compassion, "I am compassion, Itself," and pair it with its opposite of jealousy or judgment.

As you explore essential qualities and their opposites, deep residues that lie in the unconscious are liberated and bubble up into awareness. When these residues move into the light of awareness and are met with welcoming, they expand, dissolve, and reveal their Source, True Nature. As residues of stress, tension, and conflict release, they give way to feelings of relaxation, peace, and joy.

STAGE FIVE—TRANSCENDING TRUTH: AWARENESS OF THE BODY OF JOY

> *When welcoming receives everything just as it is, love blossoms and joy abounds. What*
> *wonder, astonishment, and delight.* —RICHARD MILLER

As we encounter the movement of desire, pleasure, peace, and joy, we enter into the domain governed by the *Body of Joy (anandamaya kosha)*. Evoking their associated opposites helps liberate these movements into awareness. But, ultimately, Yoga Nidra reveals that our real equanimity exists independent of all movements of emotion, belief, memory, and even joy.

Our conditioning informs us otherwise. We are taught that joy is dependent upon possession of some object: a toy, a lover, a job, a car, chocolate, or ... you name it. But true joyful equanimity is our birthright and is always present, albeit hidden behind the veil created by the dividing mind.

When we misperceive True Nature, we live identified with thoughts and emotions that inform us that contentment is dependent upon our circumstance. When you believe that you are a doer who lacks and needs to do in order to be happy, you can rest assured that you've separated from True Nature and that messengers are knocking at your door trying to inform you that you are caught in the belief that your happiness is dependent upon some object.

The search for an experience that will bring lasting joy and peace always misses the mark, as joyful equanimity is already the case. As we inquire into the Body of Joy, we discover and learn to live in joy that is devoid of any object. Then we may awaken to the realization that equanimity is always present, even in the midst of the most tumultuous and challenging circumstances.

During this phase of Yoga Nidra, we recall memories that invite joy, peace, and contentment as our embodied experience. Then we relinquish our memories and learn to recognize equanimity that is always present, that exists independent of our changing experience.

Sonia lives collapsed in her fear of being authentic. She believes, "If I just do it right I'll be loved." She distrusts herself and feels "small, worthless, and incapable." She is living a life identified with feeling separate and powerless. During Yoga Nidra, Sonia learns to rotate her attention through opposites of small-big, worthless-potent, and incapable-capable, which increases her capacity to tolerate feelings of isolation and intimacy. She learns to attune to witnessing Presence, which increases her ability to be a spacious container that welcomes every experience. As she simultaneously holds opposites of her experience, Sonia suddenly embodies the heartfelt understanding that "I'm okay, as I am." Her identity abruptly shifts from being a separate ego-I that harshly judges to an I-ness of Being in which judgments arise and are welcomed with neither reactive expression nor defensive refusing. Her self-alienation dissolves, as she feels connected to herself. Sonia begins to experience joy with her newfound self-acceptance. But even more astonishing to Sonia is when she suddenly realizes that joy and self-accepting have been with her since infancy as the equanimity of Being that has always been present. She had simply ignored this equanimity of Being because of her identification with thoughts and emotions that had occupied the foreground of her attention.

This kind of equanimity was difficult for me to comprehend at first, for I couldn't understand how joy and equanimity could co-exist alongside feelings of depression, sadness, anger, and fatigue. With doubt in hand and trust in my heart, I steadfastly practiced Yoga Nidra and realized that the ancients are right. Equanimity and joy do exist independent of whatever else is present. Yoga Nidra revealed what my mind vigorously denied. So please, have faith, persist and don't stop until you realize that peace and equanimity are the underlying fabric of your Being. Then pass on the good news.

STAGE SIX—TRUTH & SELF TRANSCENDED: AWARENESS OF THE BODY OF EGO-I

Through inquiry the mind is absorbed in silence and enlightenment naturally arises.

—YOGAVASISTHA

You are aware of everything that you experience. Sensations, emotions, thoughts, and pleasures come and go, in awareness. Yoga Nidra teaches the art of discrimination (Sanskrit: *vivekakyati*) whereby we are able to discern the difference between the objects that are coming and going in awareness, and awareness itself. Your capacity to recover this subtle discernment delivers you to the critical juncture of Yoga Nidra where you stand at the threshold of the *Body of Ego-I (asmitamaya kosha)*. At this stage we ponder the nature of this separate ego-I that we take ourselves to be, who witness and experience the myriad sensations, feelings, emotions, thoughts, and images that are coming and going in awareness.

The Great Turn of Undoing

In this phase of Yoga Nidra, you are invited to make what I call the Great Turn of Undoing wherein your attention, which has been directed outward into the objects that are in awareness, turns back upon itself and inquires into the very nature of this "I" that believes itself to be a separate witness. When the witness turns, when the one who is welcoming welcomes itself, a tremendous realization is unveiled. Your separate sense of ego-I that is identified as being a separate witness dissolves into *Being Witnessing*.

In Being, the ego-I thought cannot be sustained. It dissolves into its Source, Being. Experience this for yourself. Stop for a moment and just *BE*. Don't pay attention to any particular sensation, sound, or sight. Be open to just Being. Observe how the mind stops and thinking dissolves, absorbed in Being. This is what happens in deep sleep. Boundaries dissolve. Expansiveness unfolds. Actually "you" aren't expanding. "You" are simply returning to what you have been all along, infinite, unlimited spacious Presence.

Love, the Bodily Location of "I"

During this phase of Yoga Nidra, we learn to discriminate the difference between the changing "ego-I" that is the body, with its felt location as time-space sensation, and the "I-ness" that is Presence, which is timeless and pervasive. During Yoga Nidra, we can sub-vocally repeat "I ... I ..." while feeling where this word-sound resonates in the body. "I ... I ... " at first may be experienced in the head. Identification with thinking originates in the brain and maintains separation. But the pronoun "I" is an unusual *mantra* or sound-tool (Sanskrit: sound-tool used to transcend separation).[16] It is a tool that, when properly utilized, interrupts the mind's identification with the I-thought that creates separation.

Try the following experiment

Repeat your name sub-vocally several times (substituting your name for my name) as follows: *"I am Richard ... (pause) ... I am Richard ... (pause) ... I am Richard ... (pause) ... "* Saying your name this way reinforces your mind's identification as a separate object.

Then, drop your name and sub-vocally repeat the statement, *"I am ... (pause) ... I am ... (pause) ... I am ... (pause)."* Note the subtle shift in feeling and identity from the head and down into the heart.

Then, drop the *"am"* and sub-vocally repeat, *"I ... (pause) ... I ... (pause) ... I ... (pause)."* Then drop *"I"* and just *Be*, before mind arises and mind makes a difference. Again, note the subtle shifts into expansive openness. When used this way, the pronoun "I" is a stick that we use to stir the fire of self-inquiry that is consumed at the end in the fire of Being. All words point to Being, but "I" is a pointer par excellence.

Before thought arises in the brain and gives rise to separation, you live undivided as Being, which resonates in the body as the feeling of love that you normally associate with the heart (Sanskrit: *anahata*—unstruck sound of pure Being). Yoga Nidra develops your ability to recognize "Love" that exists independent of another. Your essence of Being or True Nature can be described as Love. As you explore the Body of Ego-I you learn to trace the feeling of "I" back to its Source and uncover Love that is your very Presence, that is present before, during, and after the I-thought, and which exists before your thinking divides the world into separate "self" and "other."

Naked Truth

When the I-thought dissolves in Love, we experience the ultimate impact of the Great Turn of Undoing where "I" is recognized in its nakedness as pure Being. Pure Being needs no separate ego-I to know Itself. Disidentification from the Body of Ego-I results in the collapse of separation. Separation is recognized as the paradox it is. Every "thing" can be metaphorically likened to objects made of gold. Gold rings, bracelets, goblets, and plates appear different in their design, but their Source is one—gold. Trees, people, animals, mountains, planets, and stars appear different, but their source is ultimately one—True Nature.

The body and mind are facets of Being. Upon disidentification from the six sheaths, Being shines forth unveiled, recognizing Itself in all of its infinite facets that reflect back its own face. We are not a separate observer, observing separate objects. This stance is a paradox, a logical absurdity, because "I" as the perceiver am not separate from "I" that is perceived. When you live this paradox without being distracted, the entire structure of separation collapses. The separative witness constructed by the mind dissolves into pure Being in which there is neither witness nor object witnessed. There is only Witnessing. There is only Perceiving. Dualistic opposites resolve into their home ground of pure Being. When subject and object dissolve, one into the other, only timeless Presence remains. Witnessing without a witness. Welcoming without a welcomer. Doing without a doer. No separation, anywhere.

Grace

Glimpses of True Nature come and go, often disappearing as quickly as they arrive. Glimpses can give way to prolonged periods of living as Being, which ultimately give way to enlightenment, the timeless instant of radical transformation in which the truth of Being fully reveals Itself. Even then, it takes time for doubt to dissolve in the truth of Being.

When you glimpse True Nature, understand that the natural tendency of your mind will still be to reassert its identity as a separate doer. But, with enlightenment, this habit is blatantly obvious. Continued inquiry dissolves the final remnants of the mind's belief in separation and uninterrupted abiding as Being becomes the norm. Then, you live the timeless realization of Yoga Nidra, which has revealed your True Nature as non-conceptual, nondual Being.

Along the way, your mind may fool itself into thinking that it is responsible for these glimpses and relapses as well as for enlightenment; that "practice makes perfect." But this is a false notion; for when we understand that everything is *Not Two* (Sanskrit: *advaita* = not two), we realize that there is no separate ego-I, or doer, who is responsible for doing any practice.[17] Everything is realized to be Grace (Sanskrit: *anugraha* = grace), which is another essential characteristic of True Nature.

Grace is everywhere for everything is Grace. Every rock and tree is Grace. Every sensation, thought, and emotion is Grace. Forgetting is Grace. Remembering is Grace. The desire and ability to awaken is Grace. And the inability to awaken is Grace, too. The child suffering is Grace. The child in joy is Grace. Peace is Grace. Even war is another face of Grace.

The recognition that everything is Grace brings with it Equanimity, which is also recognized as Grace. Grace is every situation paired with its perfect response. Embodying this understanding ends suffering, for suffering only arises when the mind defends against and pretends that Grace is so only under certain circumstances. Yoga Nidra reveals that our desire and willingness to practice, as well as the final realization of True Nature, are Grace in action. As layers of separation peel away, we recognize the "what is" of, and our true response to, each moment and realize that each is Grace.

We've heard the statement: ". . . and the Truth shall set you free." Nothing short of living in the truth of what is, works. Try every other way! You're free to try because freedom is Grace, too. In the end, when we've exhausted all avenues, we recognize how simple life is when we accept this moment, just as it is, without pretending to be other than who we are. This is Grace in action and the culmination of Yoga Nidra. What could be simpler? What could be easier? What could be more vital? Yet, throughout the world, how many understand this? So, could anything be more needed?

Let's review what has happened so far at each of these stages as we've explored the different bodies (sheaths):

- Exploring the Physical Body, we come to the conclusion that the body is not solid. It is infinite spacious vibration, without center or periphery.
- Exploring the Energy Body we realize that the body is fluid, unlimited energy.
- Exploring the Bodies of Feeling and Emotion, and Intellect, we realize that our emotions and thoughts are only passing phenomena superimposed upon a background of spacious awareness.
- Exploring the Body of Joy we realize the vastness of equanimity that exists independent of any experience.

- Exploring the Body of Ego-I, we investigate the vital questions, "Who is this 'I' that is experiencing all of these movements?" "Who is aware of these body sensations, of these flows of energy?" "Who is aware of these emotions, thoughts, and images?" In the domain of the ego-I, we inquire into the nature, substance and reality of the "I" who is aware.

STAGE SEVEN—REACHING THE SOURCE: LIVING THE NATURAL STATE

You speak as if you are here and the Self is elsewhere. The Self is here, now. You are always It.
                                                        —RAMANA MAHARSHI

The six sheaths of identification are like the emperor's new clothes.[18] Everyone pretends they exist, when in fact, they are fabrications of the mind. Separation doesn't exist, except as a projection of the mind, whose job it is to pretend that the One is actually many. Awakening from the dream of "me" reveals that every "thing" is an expression of nondual Being. Just as the facets of a diamond are not separate from the diamond, everything we see, touch, taste, hear, smell, and think is a facet of Unity. Being is the Is-ness and Suchness of every moment, the Ground out of which life springs. The essential attitude of Being is Welcoming—welcoming everything as it is, because everything is an expression of Being. Being is always welcoming itself in every moment. It cannot be otherwise. When we live knowingly as unitive Being, we feel no separation or disparity with each moment and all that life brings. Frederick Franck describes this beautifully in the story "Of Candles, Mirrors, and Wholeness."[19]

Some 1,400 years ago a brilliant woman, the Empress Wu, ruled over China. She became deeply interested in a new school of Buddhist thought, a totalistic view of the universe, which embodies one of the profoundest insights the human mind has ever attained. The Hwa Yen sages (Japanese: Kegon; Sanskrit: Avatamsaka) see the Whole, embracing all the universes as a single living organism of mutually interdependent and interpenetrating processes of becoming and un-becoming. The literature in which this cosmic vision is worked out is of extreme complexity, and so the Empress Wu decided to ask one of the founders of Hwa Yen or Kegon School, Fa Tsang (643–772 CE), if he could possibly give her a practical and simple demonstration of this cosmic interrelatedness, of the relationship of the One and the many, of God and his creatures, and of the creatures one to another.

Fa Tsang went to work and appointed one of the palace rooms so that eight large mirrors stood at the eight points of the compass. Then he placed two more mirrors, one on the ceiling and one on the floor. A candle was suspended from the ceiling in the center of the room. When the Empress entered Fa Tsang lit the candle. The Empress cried: "How marvelous! How beautiful!"

Fa Tsang pointed at the reflection of the flame in each one of the ten mirrors and said: "See, your majesty: this demonstrates the relationship of the One and the many, of God to each one of his creatures. The Empress said: "Yes, indeed, Master! And what is the relationship of each creature to the others?" Fa Tsang answered: "Just watch, your Majesty, how each mirror not only reflects the one flame in the center, each mirror also reflects the reflections of the flame in all the other mirrors, until an infinite number of flames fills them all. All these reflections are mutually identical; in a sense they are interchangeable, in another sense each one exists individually. This shows the true relationship of each being to its neighbor, to all that is! Of course I must point out, your Majesty," Fa Tsang went on, "that this is only a rough approximation and static parable of the real state of affairs in the universe—for the universe is limitless and in it all is in perpetual, multidimensional motion."

Then the Master covered one of the infinite number of reflections of the flame and showed what we are now, perhaps too late, beginning to realize in ecology—how each apparently insignificant interference affects the whole organism of our world. Kegon expresses this relationship by the formula: One in all. All in One. One in One. All in All.

Based on this insight is the Kegon term "The Great Compassionate Heart." This Great Compassionate Heart is not some mythical object. It is the quality of awareness that sees all phenomena (including of course oneself) as part of, as rising out of, Emptiness; literally remaining this Emptiness while assuming a temporal form, and finally being reabsorbed by Emptiness. It is a quality of awareness that quite naturally expresses itself in acts of deepest, yet quite unsentimental reverence and compassion for all that is, the just and the unjust, humans, animals, and even plants and stones. Is the Great Compassionate Heart perhaps what is also called the Holy Spirit?

Then Fa Tsang, in order to conclude his command performance, held up a small crystal ball and said: "Now watch, your Majesty, how all these large mirrors and all the myriad forms they reflect are mirrored in this little sphere. See how in the Ultimate Reality the infinitely small contains the infinitely large, and the infinitely large the infinitely small, without obstruction! Oh, if only I could demonstrate to you the unimpeded mutual interpenetration of time and eternity, of past, present, and future! But alas, this is a dynamic process that must be grasped on a different level."

The Hwa Yen sutra says: The incalculable eons are but one moment, and that moment is no moment, thus one sees the Reality of the Universe . . .

Hide and Seek, Lost and Found

Until we knowingly live Being, our mind will continue to play the game of "lost and found" while True Nature plays "hide and seek." But in the end we must realize that our very searching is preventing us from realizing True Nature for that, which we seek, is already what we are. The ego-I is a "hungry ghost" in search of itself. When it looks in the mirror, it sees emptiness, never realizing that Emptiness is its true form. When the I-thought dissolves in Being, we find ourselves living as Empty-Fullness—empty of self and full as everything.

I had to laugh loudly upon awakening from the "dream of me." For years I felt alone and empty, spending decades trying to remedy my plight through all means from drugs to psychotherapy and meditation. When I met my spiritual mentor, Jean Klein, his first words were, "Your very searching is taking you away."

Through his guidance, I learned to stop searching and just be. With his guidance and the support of Yoga Nidra, I began to stabilize in the equanimity of Being. And then one morning I awoke into the realization of True Nature. It was early morning around 2 a.m. when I found myself unable to sleep. I got out of bed and sat by the glass door, gazing up into the starlit nighttime sky. Suddenly, quite unexpectedly, and with no fanfare, I simply realized the underlying Essence of Being that is my True Nature and that everything is made of.

In that timeless instant, all sense of separation fell away. I recognized the truth that the ego-I is simply a thought and that everything is myself. And with that, all sense of aloneness, emptiness, and searching vanished, replaced with the irreconcilable feeling of equanimity that remains undisturbed no matter what crisis or joy is unfolding in my life. Does irritation still arise? Surely. Does fatigue and conflict still arise? Surely. But everything arises in the equanimity of Being. Of this I am convinced, as equanimity has been steadfast since that morning of awakening.

The equanimity of Being discloses an unshakable ground of stability that weathers all storms and reveals living truth and right action moment to moment. And if this realization can occur "here," I know it can occur "there" because I know it is your True Nature, too.

Your Heartfelt Prayer

As you abide in Being in this seventh stage of Yoga Nidra, with nowhere to go and nothing to do, the prayer that you began with at the beginning of your journey may re-emerge into awareness. In this moment, observe how your heartfelt prayer has changed as a result of your practice. Embody it as a heartfelt reality, how it now spontaneously arises as a resonance of truth about yourself or another. Then let it dissolve back into its home ground, Being. Affirmations come directly from True Nature and, in the end, resolve back into True Nature, and the need for them ultimately dissolves when we live the Truth of who we are.

BACK IN THE MARKETPLACE: LIVING TRUE NATURE IN EVERYDAY LIFE

Whatever the means, you must at last return to the Self; Why not abide as the Self right now?
—RAMANA MAHARSHI

Now that we have glimpsed this wondrous view from the mountaintop of Yoga Nidra, your practice continues as you learn to transpose your understanding into every moment and every relationship of your everyday life. Yoga Nidra takes you to the summit and then guides you down the mountain and back into life. Now it is time to put back on the sheaths you left behind on your way up the mountain.

The seven stages of Yoga Nidra help us take off and step away from each sheath or body of identification, the outerwear of body, mind, and senses that we had misperceived as True Nature. Yoga Nidra introduces us to the recognition of infinite spacious Being that all along is our True Nature. Now we return from where we began with the profound understanding of who we really are. As we walk back through the sheaths, putting each sheath of identification back on, we no longer need to confuse who we are with these clothes that we are wearing made of body, mind, and senses.

Facets of Unity

We now understand True Nature. That, "I am pure Awareness. I have a mind, but 'I' am not just my thoughts. I have emotions, but 'I' am not just these emotions. I have a body but 'I' am not just this body." What remains after disidentifying from body, mind, and senses is our essence of Being that is unborn and always present.

Yoga Nidra reveals that your true Essence of Being that underlies the ever-varying flow of your "personal" life, which is now realized, paradoxically, to not be "personal." Life is ultimately a paradox wherein we discover that we are non-personal Presence that gives rise to a personal self of body, mind, and senses. We are Facets of Unity. Ramana Maharshi likened the personal self as "a sliver of new moon in the noonday sky on a cloudless summer's day." While the body exists, it appears separate, yet our embodied realization is that we are non-separate Being.

Enlightened Living

Yoga Nidra reveals who we really are, initially through small glimpses. Glimpses lead to seeing through and awakening from the dream of "me." And awakening leads to enlightenment, wherein what was background, Being, moves fully foreground. As Being breaks through into the foreground, enlightenment becomes established throughout every facet of our life. With establishment, the practice of Yoga Nidra gives way to enlightened living. Here, Presence is, with no need for practice or remembering. Searching ceases, yet life continues with all of its joys and difficulties and the equanimity of Being radiantly present as the background of each moment.

At the end of Yoga Nidra, we open our eyes and step back into the world with the understanding that separation is only a product of the thinking mind. There is neither "I" nor "other" that is separate from Being. Everything is made of the same substance, the so-called external objects of the world as well as the subtle inner objects of sensation, emotion, and thought. From this perspective, there is no need to repress or refuse anything. We understand that our body and our thoughts—everything—is made of non-conceptual Being. The split-mind that divides the world into two is healed through the radical insight that Yoga Nidra reveals. Here everything is understood to be undivided Oneness. Now everything lives in Welcoming. This is the culmination of Yoga Nidra.

CHAPTER
THREE

Final Reflections

THERE ARE INFINITE forms to the practice of Yoga Nidra. As you become an accomplished practitioner, Yoga Nidra may be practiced in a matter of a few moments, or you may proceed slowly and diligently, spending an hour or more exploring and deconstructing each sheath of identification. I recommend stabilizing in one practice for a period of time.

Develop your understanding of the different stages of Yoga Nidra using the guided practices on the accompanying CD. Then experiment with your own practice. Choose one approach to body sensing and one breathing exercise. Pick one or two pairs of opposites of feeling, emotion, belief, and image. Pick one or two memories that evoke joy and peace, one approach to exploring ego-I identity and one or two qualities of True Nature to embody. Proceed slowly and dig your well deeply. The practice of Yoga Nidra takes you beyond the practice of Yoga Nidra so that in every moment you knowingly live your True Nature as Unqualified Presence of nondual Being.

Each of us is on a unique journey. While the goal is the same, our paths differ according to our stage of development. For this reason, it is important to remain mindful and attentive, adapting your practice accordingly lest it become mechanical and dull. It is important neither to impose nor deny anything. Yoga Nidra is a highly individualized practice and invites you to discover what works best for your particular needs. In this regard, please take the advice that my spiritual mentor, Jean Klein, repeatedly gave me: "Make the practice your own."

THE BODYMIND LIVES IN BEING

Don't keep Yoga Nidra just for daytime practice. Learn to practice as you fall asleep and when you awake in the middle of the night or in the morning. Waking, dreaming, and deep sleep are a continuum of consciousness. The mind only pretends they are dissimilar states. When we are awake, the mind assumes the waking state is real. When we dream, the mind assumes the dream state is real. Both waking and dreaming involve the presence of objects that are beheld in awareness. Our thinking mind is conditioned to divert attention into foreground movements and away from background awareness that is always awake as witnessing Being. Yoga Nidra invites you to be the Presence that you are during waking and sleeping without being seduced and distracted by the presence or absence of any object. True Nature needs no object to know itself. When the mind disidentifies from all movement, we stand at the threshold of True Nature, as radiant Being that transcends, yet exists in all movements.

Yoga Nidra invokes the Sleep of the Yogi wherein you are awake as unitive Being during the presence or absence of all states of consciousness. This realization is enlightenment and the culmination of Yoga Nidra where means, path, and practice merge. Here, you live free in all movements of daily life knowingly knowing yourself, all others and every "thing" as the unitive Presence that everything is; that you are. Welcome home.

Yoga Nidra Worksheet

TO PERSONALIZE YOUR practice, make several copies of these pages. Keep them in a notebook and fill in a worksheet before beginning *each* session of Yoga Nidra.

I. SETTING YOUR AFFIRMATION

Write down a positive affirmation about yourself, another, or the world around you. Write it as a statement of fact. Rather than saying, "May I be healed," or "May I be enlightened," affirm, "I am whole, healed, and healthy in this and every moment," or "My True Nature is Presence, Being."

_____

_____

_____

_____

2. THE SHEATH OF FEELING & EMOTION (MANOMAYA KOSHA)

A. Feelings

Choose two feelings and their opposites, for example, light and heavy, warm and cool.

Feeling_____ Opposite _____

Feeling_____ Opposite _____

B. Emotions

Choose two emotions and their opposites, for example, sad and happy, angry and calm.

Emotion _____ Opposite _____

Emotion _____ Opposite _____

3. THE MENTAL SHEATH (VIJÑANAMAYA KOSHA)

A. Imagery

Choose two images that engender ease and relaxation. Then choose their opposites, for example, beautiful mountain and erupting volcano, hillside of flowers and battlefield.

Image/Theme _____ Opposite _____

Image/Theme _____ Opposite _____

B. Symbol

Choose two symbols that hold meaning for you. Then choose their opposites, for example, sun and moon, circle of trusted friends and enemies at the gate.

Symbol _____ Opposite _____

Symbol _____ Opposite _____

C. Essential Qualities

Choose two essential qualities of Being and their opposites, for example, Truth and Untruth, Compassion and Arrogance; Love and Hate.

Essential Quality _____ Opposite _____

Essential Quality _____ Opposite _____

4. THE SHEATH OF JOY (ANANDAMAYA KOSHA)

Choose a memory that brings an embodiment of great joy or equanimity.

_____

_____

5. SHEATH OF EGO-I (ASMITAMAYA KOSHA)

Choose one of these exercises that explore the realm of ego-I identity.

A. Coming Home to the Self

Explore the reality of the followings statements:

"I have a body, but I am not just this body. My body manifests different sensations of health and sickness, restfulness and tiredness, calmness and agitation. But these states change. I am the unchanging awareness in which these changing sensations arise. I value my body, but I am not just this body."

"I have emotions, but I am not just these emotions. My emotions manifest different conditions from love to anger, from calmness to agitation, from joy to sorrow. But these states change. I am the unchanging awareness in which these changing emotions arise. I value my emotions, but I am not just my emotions."

"I have a mind, but I am not just my mind. My mind manifests different thoughts and images, which are constantly changing. I am the unchanging awareness in which these thoughts and images arise. I value my mind, but I am not just my mind."

"I am aware of all the changing sensations, perceptions, emotions, thoughts, and objects, which compose my body, senses, mind, and the world. I am the unchanging awareness in which all these movements arise. I am pure unchanging Awareness."

"I have a body, but I am not just my body. I have emotions, but I am not just my emotions. I have a mind, but I am not just my thoughts. What am I then? What remains after having disidentified from body, sensations, feelings, and thoughts? I am a center of pure Awareness."

B. Who Is Aware?

Body

Take a few minutes to observe your body. What are the different sensations that are present? Scanning your body, inquire gently: "Who is aware?"

Emotions

Inquire as to your emotional state. What are you feeling? If it's helpful, recall feelings from earlier events of the day or week ... Then ask yourself gently: "Who is aware? Who is aware of these feelings?"

Thoughts

Notice what you're thinking. Then inquire: "Who is aware? Who is aware of these thoughts and this thinking?"

Senses

Be aware of different smells, tastes, sounds, feelings, and images. Then gently inquire, "Who is aware? Who is aware of these perceptions? Who is aware?"

C. Self-Identification

Do not judge. View the following with the objective attitude of a scientific investigator taking an inventory.

- Become aware of body sensation. Neither change nor deny what you observe. Inquire and feel: "Who is aware of these sensations?"
- Be aware of your breathing. Inquire and feel, "Who is aware of this breathing?"
- Be aware of feelings, considering both positive and negative ones. Inquire and feel, "Who is aware of these feelings?"
- Be aware of desires, which motivate your life. Inquire and feel, "Who is aware of these desires?"
- Observe your thoughts. Witness a thought emerging. Watch it until another one takes its place, then another, and so on. If you think you are not having any thoughts, realize that this too is a thought. Inquire and feel, "Who is aware of these thoughts?"
- Observe the observer, the one who is watching sensations, feelings, desires, and thoughts. Inquire and feel, "Who is observing this observer?"
- Realize and feel the answer to every inquiry is, "I am." Feel how "I" is not solid or even a thought. "I" is a pointer to the essence of Being, in which all these realms arise and pass away. And yet, Being remains distinct from

all realms as spacious empty-full unqualified Presence. Inwardly, sense and feel the truth of this, "I am pure spacious Being, empty, yet full; Present, yet without location; everywhere, without center or periphery."

D. I Am

- Sense an object in awareness (sensation, feeling, emotion, thought, or image).
- Be aware.
- Gently, and with feeling, inquire: "Who is aware of this object?"
- Sense the answer: "I am."
- Feel where "I am" is located in the body.
- Trace the feeling from the brain, down into the heart.
- Feel the resonance of "I am" in the heart.
- Now relinquish "am." Let it drop away.
- Feel only "I ... I . . ." and where it arises in the body.
- Now drop this I-thought.
- Be one with Being, before the I-thought arises.
- Allow the observer to dissolve into Being observing.
- Allow the feeling of spacious awareness to expand simultaneously into all directions.
- Be, before the I-thought arises.
- Be, before the witness arises.
- Be, without center or periphery
- Be, before, during, and after mind arises and makes a difference.

Opposites of Feeling, Emotion, Thought, Image & Essence

THE FOLLOWING LISTS are meant as examples of opposites. Find your own or pick opposites from the category below for your personal practice of Yoga Nidra. During your practice, allow each opposite to be your embodied experience before going on to its opposite. Go back and forth several times between each pair of opposites before experiencing each pair simultaneously.

I. THE BODY OF FEELING AND EMOTION (MANOMAYA KOSHA)

A. Feelings

Awake / Sleepy

Calm / Anxious

Centered / Spacey

Comfortable / Uncomfortable

Deep / Superficial

Dry / Moist

Dull / Sharp

Floating / Sinking

Hot / Cold

Light / Heavy

Pleasurable / Painful

Relaxed / Tense

Sensitive / Numb

Spacious / Claustrophobic

Spacious / Constricted　　　　Warm / Cool
Strong / Weak

B. Emotions

Aggressive / Passive　　　　　Loving / Hateful
Approving / Disapproving　　　Peaceful / Enraged
Assured / Perplexed　　　　　Potent / Impotent
Boisterous / Mellow　　　　　Powerful / Helpless
Calm / Agitated　　　　　　　Proud / Ashamed
Composed / Worried　　　　　Responsive / Apathetic
Confident / Insecure　　　　　Safe / Abandoned
Cooperative / Competitive　　 Safe / Threatened
Delighted / Disgusted　　　　 Satisfied / Frustrated
Domineering / Meek　　　　　Secure / Apprehensive
Empathic / Indifferent　　　　Sensitive / Numb
Fearless / Frightened　　　　　Tender / Violent
Flexible / Obstinate　　　　　 Tolerant / Contemptuous
Generous / Resentful　　　　　Trusting / Suspicious
Grateful / Ungrateful　　　　　Unafraid / Anxious
Happy / Sad　　　　　　　　　Unreserved / Shy
Helpful / Uncooperative　　　　Vital / Exhausted
Innocent / Guilty　　　　　　 Vulnerable / Invulnerable
Interested / Bored

2. THE BODY OF INTELLECT (VIJÑANAMAYA KOSHA)

A. Images and Symbols

Allow each image to be evocative on all levels of feeling, emotion, and imagination.

A circle of trusted friends

Birds flying

Burning candle

Cat reposing

Cave leading down into the ground

Coffin

Cross

Dark sky

Tunnel

Dead body

Dying person

Endless desert

Frail old man

Frail old woman

Horse running

Human skeleton

Ocean

Space

Knife

Naked body

People at war

People shouting

Smiling Buddha

Sun rising in the sky

Sun setting in the sky

Torrential rain

Waves breaking on a beach

Well going down into the ground

Clouds floating across the sky

Wise old man

Wise old woman

Yogi in meditation

B. Themes

Moving through a tunnel

Performing an asana practice

Traveling down a river

Traveling down an opening

Traveling down into the ocean depths

Traveling into the future

Traveling into the past

Traveling up a mountain

Traveling up into the sky

Walking along the ocean

Walking in the desert

C. Essential Qualities of Presence

Experience the following essential qualities of Presence. Allow each quality to evoke feelings, emotions, thoughts, images, and memories. Allow all channels of perception to participate in the experience: seeing, hearing, tasting, smelling, touching, and thinking.

Authentic	Intelligent
Awake	Intimate
Aware	Joyful
Being	Loving
Compassionate	Peaceful
Creative	Powerful
Empathic	Present
Empty	Spacious
Expansive	Welcoming
Full	

Resources for Supporting Your Practice

SO, YOU'VE READ this book, listened to the CD, and are now thinking, "What's next?" "Is there someone I can talk to or consult with regarding my practice?" "Where do I go from here?"

CONTACT THE AUTHOR

I offer private consultations, mentoring, seminars, workshops, and retreats during which I provide basic instruction and advanced trainings in Yoga Nidra for beginners through advanced trainees and teachers. I also train teachers throughout the United States and Canada. Please visit my web site, send me an e-mail, or call my office for the location of a nearby training or a listing of teachers in your area.

ADVANCED PRACTICES

Infinite Awakening: The Principles and Practice of Yoga Nidra, a set of five recorded sessions on Yoga Nidra, is available through my web site and office. These recordings consist of a 35-minute introduction and five 40-minute practice sessions covering in-depth explorations of the stages of Yoga Nidra. I continually produce practice and training materials on Yoga Nidra. Please contact my office directly for further details.

Explorations in Stillness
PO Box 1673
Sebastopol CA 95473
(707) 876-3380 / www.nondual.com / info@nondual.com

TRADITIONAL TRAINING

Yoga centers throughout the world offer training in Yoga Nidra as part of their curriculum. Teachers/training facilities I recommend are:

Swami Veda Bharati

Swami Veda has spent over five decades providing spiritual guidance around the world. In 1969, he met his Spiritual Master, Swami Rama, who initiated him into the path of Dhyana Yoga. Swami Veda is well versed in the scriptures of all religions, understands seventeen languages, and is familiar with all known meditative traditions. He lectures and offers retreats, workshops, and trainings worldwide. Yoga Nidra lies at the heart of his teachings. For further studies, please contact:

In the United States
The Meditation Center
631 University Ave. NE
Minneapolis MN 55413
612-379-2386 / www.bindu.org / info@themeditationcenter.org

In India
Swami Rama Sadhaka Grama
Virpur Khurd Village
Virbhadra Road P.O. Pashulok
Rishikesh UA, India 249203
+91 135-2450093, 2450596 / www.bindu.org / sadhaka_grama@yahoo.com

Paramhamsa Satyananda

Satyananda studied Tantric forms of Yoga from an early age, finding his calling at age nineteen when he met his guru, Swami Sivananda of Rishikesh, India, who initiated him into swamihood in 1947. In 1963, Satyananda established the Bihar School of Yoga in Bihar, India. First published in 1976, Satyananda's book, *Yoga Nidra*, continues to be a premier writing in the field of Yoga Nidra. For further studies contact:

Bihar School of Yoga
PO Rikhia
Dist. Deoghar
Jharkhand India 814 112
Tel: +91-6432 232870 / Fax: +91-6432 230670 / www.satyananda.net

Swami Janakananda

Founder of the Scandinavian Yoga and Meditation School, Janakananda is a student of Swami Satyananda, with whom he trained in India. Janakananda and his teachers provide trainings and support throughout Europe in the practice of Yoga Nidra. They also offer CDs and books to support your practice.

Scandinavian Yoga and Meditation School
S-34013 Hamneda, Sweden
Tel: +46 372 550 63 / Fax: +46 372 550 36 / www.scand-yoga.org

Rod Stryker

Founder of Pure Yoga, Rod is a student of Pandit Rajmani Tigunait, Ph.D., and a teacher in the lineage of the Swami Rama of the Himalayas. Rod offers trainings and support throughout the United States in the practice of Yoga Nidra. He is the author of CDs and books, which are designed to support your practice including *Relax into Greatness,* which offers a long and short version of Yoga Nidra.

Pure Yoga
1351 Westwood Blvd, #120
Los Angeles CA 90024
(310) 745-1071 / www.pureyoga.com

References

Barks, Coleman & Moyne, John, *Unseen Rain,* Threshold Books, VT, 1984.

Bly, Robert, *The Kabir Book,* Beacon Press, Boston, 1971.

Feuerstein, Georg, *Encyclopedic Dictionary of Yoga,* Paragon House, 1990.

Franck, Frederick, *The Book of Angelus Silesius,* Bear & Co., Santa Fe, 1985.

Gazzaniga, Michael, *The Mind's Past,* University of California Press, Berkeley, 1998.

Jenny, Hans, *Cymatics,* Vol I & II, Basilius Press, Germany, 1967 & 1972.

Klein, Jean, *Transmission of the Flame,* Third Millennium Publications, Santa Barbara, 1990.

Klein, Jean, *I Am,* Third Millennium Publications, Santa Barbara, 1989.

Klein, Jean, *Who Am I,* Third Millennium Publications, Santa Barbara, 1988.

Klein, Jean, *The Ease of Being,* Third Millennium Publications, Santa Barbara, 1984.

Kornfield, Jack, *After the Ecstasy, the Laundry,* Bantam, NY, 2000.

Kohn, Sherab Chodzin, *The Awakened One: A Life of the Buddha,* Shambhala, Boston, 1994.

Liberman, Jacob, *Light Medicine of the Future,* Bear & Company, NM, 1990.

Libet, Benjamin, *Mind Time: The Temporal Factor in Consciousness,* Harvard University Press, Harvard, A, 2004 (p. 47, line 42).

Maharshi, Ramana, *The Spiritual Teachings of Ramana Maharshi,* Shambhala, 1988.

Miller, Richard C., *Infinite Awakening: The Principles and Practice of Yoga Nidra Audiotapes,* Anahata Press, PO Box 1673, Sebastopol, CA 95473, 2001.

Mishra, Rammurti S., *Fundamentals of Yoga: A Handbook of Theory, Practice, and Application,* Julian Press, 1979.

Mishra, Rammurti S., *Yoga Sutras: The Textbook of Yoga Psychology,* Anchor Press, NY, 1973.

Niranjanananda, Swami, *Prana, Pranayama, Prana Vidya,* Bihar School of Yoga, 1994.

Rama, Swami, *Exercise without Movement,* Himalayan Institute, Honesdale, PA, 1984.

Rama, Swami, *Joints and Glands Exercises,* Himalayan Institute, Honesdale, PA, 1982.

Reps, Paul & Senzaki, Nyogen, *Zen Flesh, Zen Bones,* Tuttle Publishing, Boston, 1985.

Satyananda, Swami, *Yoga Nidra,* Bihar School of Yoga, India 1976.

Satyananda, Swami, *Meditation from the Tantras,* Bihar School of Yoga, 1974.

Venkatesananda, Swami, *Enlightened Living: A New Interpretative Translation of the Yoga Sutra of Maharshi Patañjali,* Anahata Press, Sebastopol, CA, 1999.

Weber, Gary, *You Don't Exist, You Are Everything: Yoga, Zen, and Advaita Vedanta for Nondual Awakening,* private manuscript, 2005, www.nittanydharma.org/nondual.

Wei Wu Wei, *Open Secret,* Hong Kong University Press, Hong Kong, 1982.

Readings Particular to Nondual Kashmir Shaivism

Hughes, John, *Self Realization in Kashmir Shaivism,* SUNY, NY, 1994.

Odier, Daniel, *Desire: The Tantric Path to Awakening,* Inner Traditions, VT, 2001.

Singh, Jaideva, *Pratyabhijñahrdayam: The Secret of Self-Recognition,* Motilal, India 1998.

Singh, Jaideva, *Siva Sutras: The Yoga of Supreme Identity.* Motilal, India 1998.

Singh, Jaideva, *Spanda Karikas: The Divine Creative Pulsation,* Motilal, India 1994.

Singh, Jaideva, *Vijñanabhairav: The Yoga of Delight, Wonder & Astonishment,* Motilal, India 1979.

Notes

1 *Bhagavad Gita,* 2:61-66. Author's translation.

2 Wu Wei Wu, *Open Secret.*

3 These include the nondual teachings of *Trika-Shasana* as found in the revelatory Shiva Sutras; Tantra in such texts as the Mahanirvana; Vedanta in writings such as the *Mandukya, Taittiriya Upanisads* and *Tripura Rahasya;* and the teachings of Yoga as found in *Yogataravali*and the *Yoga Sutra of Patañjali* with its emphasis on *pratyahara* (Sanskrit: *restoration of the senses to their natural functioning*) wherein the mind's propensity to identify with its projections is transcended and we realize our true nature as unitive Being.

4 See References for works by these authors.

5 In particular, I offer profound gratitude and thanks to Laura Cummings, J. Krishnamurti, Bikram Choudhury, Joel Kramer, Da Free John, Swami Bua, B.K.S. Iyengar, T.K.V. Desikachar, Dada, Nisargadatta Maharaj, Ramesh Balsekar, Ramana Maharshi, and my spiritual sat guru, Jean Klein.

6 The *Yoga Sutra of Patañjali* utilizes the word, *nirodha,* to describe True Nature as "Pure Being" or "Stillness." which we are always being, whether we realize it or not. *Yogash Citta Vritti Nirodhah: Yoga happens when we realize our True Nature as that Stillness or Pure Being, which is always present, whether the movements of consciousness are present or absent* (chapter I, verse 2, author's translation).

7 Werner Heisenberg, the founder of quantum mechanics stated in his 1927 uncertainty paper that, *"The more the position of an object is determined the less its momentum is known, and vice versa."* He uncovered what Yoga Nidra has affirmed

for centuries, that as an observer we are not separate from what we observe. The observer and object are actually one, not two. What appears as a solid universe is actually empty space.

8 To further your understanding, please read Gazzaniga, *The Mind's Past*.

9 Author's private correspondence with Alicia Higham. Used with her permission.

10 Gazzaniga, *The Mind's Past*, pg. 71.

11 *Yoga Sutra of Patañjali*, Chapter II, verse 17.

12 See the *Spandakarika*.

13 See Swami Veda Baharti: www.bindu.org/svbresearchpage1.html; Swami Rama: Exercise without Movement; Swami Satyananda: *Yoga Nidra*.

14 Prana (Sanskrit) literally means, "breathing forth the vibratory force that underlies all manifestation." See Feuerstein, *Encyclopedic Dictionary of Yoga*.

15 *Unseen Rain*, Coleman Barks, quatrain 158.

16 Sanskrit: *man-* "to think" and *tra-* "instrumentality" (Feuerstein, 1990). Mantra is the instrument of sound that is used to transcend the thinking mind and heal the myth of separation.

17 If we affirm that everything is One, its opposite co-arises, that there are "two." But "not two" has no opposite and refers directly to our True Nature.

18 *Emperor'sNew Clothes* by Hans Christian Andersen, www.broadviewpress.com/tales/emperorsclothes.htm

19 Franck, *The Book of Angelus Silesius*. Permission granted by Frederick Franck (© 1976 Frederick Franck) by permission of Alfred A. Knopf, a division of Random House, Inc.

RICHARD MILLER, PH.D., has traversed the path of nondualism ever since the universe revealed its truth of oneness while he was lying in a sand trap gazing into the starlit sky at the ripe age of 13. Along the way he studied Taoism and Chinese Medicine, co-authoring *The Book of Internal Exercises* and volunteering his acupuncture skills at a village clinic while studying Yoga in India. He holds a BS in psychology (1970), an MA in communication (1975) and a Ph.D. in clinical psychology (1987). Many gifted teachers have influenced him including Laura Cummings, T.K.V. Desikachar, Ramesh Balsekar, and Suzanne Segal. Following a series of awakenings that began in childhood, all sense of separation fell away while studying with his spiritual mentor, Jean Klein. Richard experiences this awakening as always fresh, always alive, always opening to itself. In private practice since 1972, he continues today having "conversations" with people interested in awakening to their nondual true nature.

Richard is recognized as a leading force in the field of Yoga, honored by *Yoga Journal* and featured in *American Yoga* (Barnes & Noble). Richard co-founded The International Association of Yoga Therapy and was founding editor of its professional journal. He has authored numerous articles including "Welcoming All That Is" in *Paragon's* The Sacred Mirror: Nondual Wisdom and Psychotherapy. His current interests include bringing the meditative process of Yoga Nidra to public attention, writing books on nondual meditation, and providing translations of traditional Sanskrit texts of Yoga and Nonduality. More than anything Richard enjoys hosting retreats where people gather to his creative way of teaching with its focus on awakening and embodying true nature in everyday life. He can be contacted through his web site, www.nondual.com.

Sounds True was founded with a clear vision: to disseminate spiritual wisdom. Located in Boulder, Colorado, Sounds True publishes teaching programs that are designed to educate, uplift, and inspire. With more than 600 titles available, we work with many of the leading spiritual teachers, thinkers, healers, and visionary artists of our time.

For a free catalog or for more information on audio programs by Richard Miller, please contact Sounds True via the World Wide Web at www.soundstrue.com, call us toll free at 800-333-9185, or write:

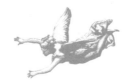

The Sounds True Catalog
PO Box 8010
Boulder CO 80306